T0263617

The Evolving Role of Therapeutic Endoscopy in Patients with Chronic Liver Diseases

Editor

ANDRES F. CARRION

CLINICS IN
LIVER DISEASE

www.liver.theclinics.com

Consulting Editor
NORMAN GITLIN

February 2022 • Volume 26 • Number 1

ELSEVIER

1600 John F. Kennedy Boulevard • Suite 1800 • Philadelphia, Pennsylvania, 19103-2899

http://www.theclinics.com

CLINICS IN LIVER DISEASE Volume 26, Number 1
February 2022 ISSN 1089-3261, ISBN-13: 978-0-323-84882-4

Editor: Kerry Holland
Developmental Editor: Ann Gielou M. Posedio

© **2022 Elsevier Inc. All rights reserved.**

This periodical and the individual contributions contained in it are protected under copyright by Elsevier, and the following terms and conditions apply to their use:

Photocopying

Single photocopies of single articles may be made for personal use as allowed by national copyright laws. Permission of the Publisher and payment of a fee is required for all other photocopying, including multiple or systematic copying, copying for advertising or promotional purposes, resale, and all forms of document delivery. Special rates are available for educational institutions that wish to make photocopies for non-profit educational classroom use. For information on how to seek permission visit www.elsevier.com/permissions or call: (+44) 1865 843830 (UK)/ (+1) 215 239 3804 (USA).

Derivative Works

Subscribers may reproduce tables of contents or prepare lists of articles including abstracts for internal circulation within their institutions. Permission of the Publisher is required for resale or distribution outside the institution. Permission of the Publisher is required for all other derivative works, including compilations and translations (please consult www.elsevier.com/permissions).

Electronic Storage or Usage

Permission of the Publisher is required to store or use electronically any material contained in this periodical, including any article or part of an article (please consult www.elsevier.com/permissions). Except as outlined above, no part of this publication may be reproduced, stored in a retrieval system or transmitted in any form or by any means, electronic, mechanical, photocopying, recording or otherwise, without prior written permission of the Publisher.

Notice

No responsibility is assumed by the Publisher for any injury and/or damage to persons or property as a matter of products liability, negligence or otherwise, or from any use or operation of any methods, products, instructions or ideas contained in the material herein. Because of rapid advances in the medical sciences, in particular, independent verification of diagnoses and drug dosages should be made.

Although all advertising material is expected to conform to ethical (medical) standards, inclusion in this publication does not constitute a guarantee or endorsement of the quality or value of such product or of the claims made of it by its manufacturer.

Clinics in Liver Disease (ISSN 1089-3261) is published quarterly by Elsevier Inc., 360 Park Avenue South, New York, NY 10010-1710. Months of issue are February, May, August, and November. Business and Editorial Offices: 1600 John F. Kennedy Blvd., Ste. 1800, Philadelphia, PA 19103-2899. Customer Service Office: 3251 Riverport Lane, Maryland Heights, MO 63043. Periodicals postage paid at New York, NY and additional mailing offices. Subscription prices are $329.00 per year (U.S. individuals), $100.00 per year (U.S. student/resident), $782.00 per year (U.S. institutions), $421.00 per year (international individuals), $200.00 per year (international student/resident), $813.00 per year (international instituitions), $382.00 per year (Canadian individuals), $100.00 per year (Canadian student/resident), and $813.00 per year (Canadian institutions). Foreign air speed delivery is included in all Clinics subscription prices. All prices are subject to change without notice. **POSTMASTER:** Send address changes to Clinics in Liver Disease, Elsevier Health Sciences Division, Subscription Customer Service, 3251 Riverport Lane, Maryland Heights, MO 63043. **Customer Service: Telephone: 1-800-654-2452 (U.S. and Canada); 314-447-8871 (outside U.S. and Canada). Fax: 314-447-8029. E-mail: journalscustomer service-usa@elsevier.com (for print support); journalsonlinesupport-usa@elsevier.com (for online support).**

Reprints. For copies of 100 or more of articles in this publication, please contact the Commercial Reprints Department, Elsevier Inc., 360 Park Avenue South, New York, NY 10010-1710. Tel.: 212-633-3874; Fax: 212-633-3820; E-mail: reprints@elsevier.com.

Clinics in Liver Disease is covered in MEDLINE/PubMed (Index Medicus), Science Citation Index Expanded, Journal Citation Reports/Science Edition, and Current Contents/Clinical Medicine.

Contributors

CONSULTING EDITOR

NORMAN GITLIN, MD, FRCP (LONDON), FRCPE (EDINBURGH), FAASLD, FACP, FACG
Head of Hepatology, Southern California Liver Centers, San Clemente, California, USA

EDITOR

ANDRES F. CARRION, MD
Associate Professor of Clinical Medicine, Division of Digestive Health and Liver Diseases, University of Miami Miller School of Medicine, Miami, Florida, USA

AUTHORS

SUNIL AMIN, MD, MPH
Division of Digestive Health and Liver Diseases, Department of Medicine, University of Miami, Miami, Florida, USA

MONIQUE T. BARAKAT, MD, PhD
Division of Gastroenterology, Stanford University School of Medicine, Stanford, California, USA

KALYAN RAM BHAMIDIMARRI, MD, MPH, FACG, FAASLD
Division of Digestive Health and Liver Diseases, University of Miami Miller School of Medicine, Miami, Florida, USA

JOHN J. BRANDABUR, MD
Digestive Health Institute, Swedish Medical Center, Seattle, Washington, USA

MARCO A. BUSTAMANTE-BERNAL, MD
Clinical Faculty, Division of Gastroenterology and Hepatology, Texas Tech University Health Sciences Center, El Paso, Texas, USA

CHRISTOPHER J. CARLSON, MD
Digestive Health Institute, Swedish Medical Center, Seattle, Washington, USA

LUIS O. CHAVEZ, MD
Fellow, Division of Gastroenterology and Hepatology, Texas Tech University Health Sciences Center, El Paso, Texas, USA

EMMANUEL CORONEL, MD
Department of Gastroenterology, Hepatology, and Nutrition, The University of Texas MD Anderson Cancer Center, Houston, Texas, USA

MARTIN CORONEL, MD
Department of Gastroenterology, Hepatology, and Nutrition, The University of Texas MD Anderson Cancer Center, Houston, Texas, USA

AMEESH DEV, MD
School of Medicine, University of Texas Health San Antonio, San Antonio, Texas, USA

CYRUS V. EDELSON, MD
Department of Medicine, Division of Gastroenterology, Brooke Army Medical Center, Houston, Texas, USA

SHERIF ELHANAFI, MD
Assistant Professor of Medicine, Division of Gastroenterology and Hepatology, Texas Tech University Health Sciences Center, El Paso, Texas, USA

JUSTIN J. FORDE, MD, MS
Division of Digestive Health and Liver Diseases, University of Miami Miller School of Medicine, Miami, Florida, USA

LAWRENCE S. FRIEDMAN, MD
The Anton R. Fried, MD, Chair, Department of Medicine, Newton-Wellesley Hospital, Newton, Massachusetts, USA; Assistant Chief of Medicine, Massachusetts General Hospital, Professor of Medicine, Harvard Medical School, Professor of Medicine, Tufts University School of Medicine, Boston, Massachusetts, USA

MOHIT GIROTRA, MD, FACP
Consultant Gastroenterologist and Therapeutic Endoscopist, Digestive Health Institute, Swedish Medical Center, Seattle, Washington, USA

TARA KEIHANIAN, MD, MPH
Division of Gastroenterology, Baylor College of Medicine, Houston, Texas, USA

JEFFREY H. LEE, MD, MPH
Department of Gastroenterology, Hepatology, and Nutrition, The University of Texas MD Anderson Cancer Center, Houston, Texas, USA

JAY LUTHER, MD
MGH Alcohol Liver Center, Division of Gastroenterology, Department of Medicine, Massachusetts General Hospital, Assistant Professor of Medicine, Harvard Medical School, Boston, Massachusetts, USA

ISHAAN K. MADHOK, MD
Resident Physician, Department of Internal Medicine, University of Florida, Gainesville, Florida, USA

ANTONIO MENDOZA LADD, MD
Associate Professor of Medicine, Division of Gastroenterology and Hepatology, Texas Tech University Health Sciences Center, El Paso, Texas, USA

RAJNISH MISHRA, MD
Digestive Health Institute, Swedish Medical Center, Seattle, Washington, USA

CHRIS MOREAU, BSBME
Department of Medicine, Division of Gastroenterology, University of Texas Health San Antonio, San Antonio, Texas, USA

AHMAD NAKSHABANDI, MD
Department of Gastroenterology and Hepatology, MedStar Georgetown University Hospital, Washington, DC, USA

JOSE M. NIETO, DO, AGAF, FACP, FACG, FASGE
Chair, Advanced Therapeutic Endoscopy Center, Borland Groover, Jacksonville, Florida, USA

ROBERTO OLEAS, MD
Research Fellow, Instituto Ecuatoriano de Enfermedades Digestivas, Guayaquil, Ecuador

MOHAMED O. OTHMAN, MD
Chief, Gastroenterology Section, BSLMC, William T. Butler Endowed Chair for Distinguished Faculty, Professor of Medicine, Gastroenterology and Hepatology Section, Baylor College of Medicine, Houston, Texas, USA

NASIM PARSA, MD
Advanced Fellow, Esophageal Diseases, Division of Gastroenterology and Hepatology, Mayo Clinic, Scottsdale, Arizona, USA

SANDEEP N. PATEL, DO
Clinical Associate Professor, Department of Medicine, Division of Gastroenterology, University of Texas Health San Antonio, San Antonio, Texas, USA

DAVID J. RESTREPO, MD
Department of Medicine, Division of Internal Medicine, University of Texas Health San Antonio, San Antonio, Texas, USA

CARLOS ROBLES-MEDRANDA, MD
Head of the Endoscopy Division, Instituto Ecuatoriano de Enfermedades Digestivas, Guayaquil, Ecuador

MANASI RUNGTA, BS
Gastroenterology and Hepatology Section, Baylor College of Medicine, Houston, Texas, USA

SHREYAS SALIGRAM, MD, MRCP (UK), FACG, FASGE
Clinical Assistant Professor, Department of Medicine, Division of Gastroenterology, University of Texas Health San Antonio, San Antonio, Texas, USA

HARI SAYANA, MD
Clinical Assistant Professor, Department of Medicine, Division of Gastroenterology, University of Texas Health San Antonio, San Antonio, Texas, USA

ENRICO O. SOUTO, MD
Assistant Professor of Clinical Medicine, Division of Digestive Health and Liver Diseases, University of Miami Miller School of Medicine, Miami, Florida, USA

SOORAJ TEJASWI, MD, MSPH
Division of Gastroenterology, Sutter Medical Group, Davis, California, USA

SHYAM VEDANTAM, DO
Department of Medicine, University of Miami, Miami, Florida, USA

MARC J. ZUCKERMAN, MD
Professor of Medicine, Division of Gastroenterology and Hepatology, Texas Tech University Health Sciences Center, El Paso, Texas, USA

Contents

Management of coagulopathy in patients with advanced liver disease undergoing therapeutic endoscopic procedures is complex. Improvements in the understanding of hemostasis at a physiologic level have highlighted the inaccuracy of currently available clinical tests, like platelet count and prothrombin time, in estimating hemostasis in patients with cirrhosis. With identification of novel factors that contribute to bleeding risk in patients with cirrhosis, there is a dearth of clinical trial data that account for all potentially relevant factors and that examine interventions to reduce bleeding risk. Precise recommendations regarding transfusion strategies based on hemostatic test results in patients with cirrhosis are impractical.

Endoscopic mucosal resection and dissection are advanced endoscopic procedures that have proven essential for resecting premalignant and early malignant lesions throughout the gastrointestinal tract. Over time, these procedures have proven to play a key role in avoiding more invasive surgical approaches and thus decrease overall mortality. However, the success of these procedures does come with a slightly increased risk of adverse events such as bleeding and perforation. In this article, we review the literature for reported adverse events, specifically in the cirrhotic population. This article also discusses experts' opinions on approaches taken to perform these procedures with acceptable risks.

Acute variceal bleeding is a complication of portal hypertension, usually due to cirrhosis, with high morbidity and mortality. There are 3 scenarios for endoscopic treatment of esophageal varices: prevention of first variceal bleed, treatment of active variceal bleed, and prevention of rebleeding. Patients with cirrhosis should be screened for esophageal varices. Recommended endoscopic therapy for acute variceal bleeding is endoscopic variceal banding. Although banding is the first-choice treatment, sclerotherapy may have a role. Treatment with Sengstaken-Blakemore tube or self-expanding covered metallic esophageal stent can be used for acute variceal bleeding refractory to standard pharmacologic and endoscopic therapy.

Gastric variceal bleeding has a high mortality. Endoscopic cyanoacrylate injection is the standard therapy; however, rebleeding and unexpected adverse events, such as injection sites ulcers and distal glue embolisms, are pitfalls of this therapy. Endoscopic ultrasound (EUS)-guided endovascular therapies offer a safer and more practical alternative for the treatment of gastric varices. EUS-guided combined therapy with coiling and cyanoacrylate injection is the most promising alternative with high obliteration rates and fewer adverse events reported. The authors reviewed the latest available data for all endoscopic therapies proposed for the management of gastric varices in patients with chronic liver disease.

Cholestatic liver diseases (CLDs) occur as a result of bile duct injury, emanating into duct obstruction and bile stasis. Advances in radiological imaging in the last decade has replaced endoscopic retrograde cholangiopancreatography (ERCP) as the first diagnostic tool, except in certain groups of patients, such as those with ischemic cholangiopathy (IsC) or early stages of primary sclerosing cholangitis (PSC). ERCP provides an opportunity for targeted tissue acquisition for histopathological evaluation and carries a diverse therapeutic profile to restore bile flow. The aim of this review article is to appraise the diagnostic and therapeutic roles of ERCP in CLDs.

Indeterminate biliary strictures are defined as a narrowing of the bile duct that cannot be differentiated as malignant or benign after performing cross-sectional imaging and an ERCP. Identifying the etiology of a bile duct stricture is the single most important step in determining whether a complex and potentially morbid surgical resection is warranted. Due to this diagnostic and therapeutic dilemma, new technologies, laboratory tests, and procedures are emerging to solve this problem.

Biliary complications are often referred to as the Achilles' heel of liver transplantation (LT). The most common of these complications include strictures, and leaks. Prompt diagnosis and management is key for preservation of the transplanted organ. Unfortunately, a number of factors can lead to delays in diagnosis and make adequate treatment a challenge. Innovations in advanced endoscopic techniques have increased non-surgical options for these complications and in many cases is the preferred approach.

If endoscopic retrograde cholangiopancreatography (ERCP) fails in cases of biliary obstruction and jaundice, percutaneous drains have been traditionally the current second-line option. Endoscopic ultrasonography-guided biliary drainage (EUS-BD) with choledocoduodenostomy or hepaticogastrostomy is alternative modality that have shown equivalent or better technical and clinical success compared with percutaneous drainage. Similarly, EUS-guided gallbladder drainage has emerged as a therapeutic option in acute cholecystitis as well. Furthermore, EUS-BD avoids some of the pitfalls of percutaneous drainage. Current research in EUS-BD involves optimizing devices to improve technical and clinical success. In centers with advanced endoscopists trained in these procedures, EUS-BD is an excellent second-line modality.

Cholangiocarcinoma (CCA) is the most common neoplasm of the biliary tract. The biological behavior and prognosis of CCA vary depending on the tumor's location in the biliary tree, dictating a different diagnostic, and treatment approach. Establishing a diagnosis of CCA remains a challenge and up to 20% of biliary strictures can yield indeterminate results, despite extensive evaluation. Endoscopic ultrasound (EUS) has become an effective diagnostic tool, as it provides high-quality images of the bile duct and allows for the sampling of strictures in the same plane of view. In this chapter, we explore the utility of EUS as a diagnostic and staging tool for biliary cancers.

Endoscopic ultrasound-guided liver biopsy (EUS-LB) has emerged as a safe and effective alternative to percutaneous and trans-jugular approaches for hepatic tissue acquisition. It has shown superior diagnostic yield for the targeted approach of focal lesions, less sampling variability, improved patient comfort, and safety profile. These advantages have contributed to the increased use of EUS-LB as a technique for obtaining liver tissue. In this review, we provide an update on the recent evidence of EUS-LB for the evaluation of liver disease.

Obesity and its associated comorbidities are rapidly increasing in the US population. Therefore, metabolic associated fatty liver disease (MAFLD),

CLINICS IN LIVER DISEASE

SERIES OF RELATED INTEREST

Gastroenterology Clinics of North America
https://www.gastro.theclinics.com

THE CLINICS ARE AVAILABLE ONLINE!
Access your subscription at:
www.theclinics.com

Preface

Through the Scope Hepatobiliary Interventions in Patients with Liver Diseases: Minimizing Risks and Improving Outcomes

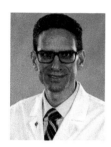

Andres F. Carrion, MD
Editor

The use of advanced endoscopic techniques in the field of hepatology has rapidly expanded over the last decade. Traditionally, endoscopy in patients with chronic liver disease was limited to screening/surveillance of gastroesophageal varices and colorectal polyps as well as endoscopic interventions for prophylaxis and treatment of acute variceal hemorrhage. Interventions such as endoscopic retrograde cholangio-pancreatography (ERCP) have become standard of care for various hepatobiliary disorders and permit minimally invasive management, reducing the need for surgical and percutaneous interventions. ERCP evolved from a diagnostic to a therapeutic intervention, and ongoing improvements of accessories and novel devices continue to pave the road for increased therapeutic capabilities, even in highly complex cases. Biliary complications, once considered the *Achilles heel* of liver transplantation, can nowadays be treated successfully with ERCP in most patients. Balloon dilatation and incremental plastic stenting has been the treatment of choice for anastomotic biliary strictures in liver transplant recipients, obviating surgical reintervention. Novel therapeutic strategies, such as sequential plastic stent addition and using fully covered self-expandable metal stents, offer attractive alternatives to frequent plastic stent replacement with comparable outcomes. Single-operator cholangioscopy has dramatically improved over the past decade and now offers digital imaging on an extremely versatile platform, which has greatly increased the diagnostic yield of ERCP in the evaluation of biliary strictures by permitting accurate evaluation of vascular patterns in addition to providing image-guided sampling and therapeutic capabilities.

Clin Liver Dis 26 (2022) xiii–xv
https://doi.org/10.1016/j.cld.2021.09.003
1089-3261/22/© 2021 Published by Elsevier Inc.

Endoscopic ultrasound (EUS) has also evolved from a purely image-based diagnostic procedure to an image-guided tissue sampling and therapeutic intervention. Although the endosonographic characteristics of certain lesions are important to differentiate benign versus malignant behavior, EUS-guided fine needle aspiration and fine needle biopsy permit histologic confirmation. EUS-guided liver biopsy is a clear example of refinement of an old technique and appropriate usage of technology to improve histologic samples and potentially decrease adverse events. The use of EUS guidance to obtain core liver biopsies has several theoretic advantages, at least compared with the percutaneous route. EUS provides real-time imaging with Doppler capability, and the needle travels only a very short distance to access both liver lobes, the latter being a significant advantage in obese patients. Improvements in core needles and suction/actuation techniques have dramatically improved the quality of tissue samples and the histologic yield. Furthermore, EUS-guided liver biopsy can be performed during the same session as esophagogastroduodenoscopy (EGD) for screening for gastroesophageal varices, and recovery time is significantly shorter than percutaneous techniques.

The applications of therapeutic EUS in patients with liver diseases continue to evolve. EUS-guided biliary drainage and endovascular access are some of the most exciting areas. Up until recently, percutaneous cholecystostomy drains were the main alternative for gallbladder drainage in patients with acute cholecystitis at high risk for surgery. Traditionally, most patients with decompensated liver disease and acute cholecystitis have been treated with percutaneous cholecystostomy drains, which are associated with significant adverse events and markedly reduced quality of life. Furthermore, there is usually no clear endpoint for these drains in this population. EUS-guided gallbladder drainage offers a safe, effective, and minimally invasive alternative to percutaneous cholecystostomy with improved quality of life. Although endoscopic therapy for esophageal varices is highly effective for prophylaxis and treatment of active hemorrhage, gastric varices have been difficult to treat endoscopically. Some centers offer endoscopic therapy for gastric varices with cyanoacrylate "glue" injection; however, there are important limitations to this therapy. EUS-guided endovascular coiling is an emerging technique associated with excellent technical and clinical success as well as a reassuring safety profile. Furthermore, a combination of EUS-guided coiling and glue injection appears to be an excellent therapeutic option for actively bleeding gastric varices in patients with severely decompensated chronic liver disease deemed to be at high risk for transjugular intrahepatic portosystemic shunt placement. Although not a therapeutic intervention but rather having important diagnostic and prognostic implications, EUS-guided portal pressure measurement presents an exciting opportunity to *directly* measure portal pressures in clinical practice. Selected centers, particularly in Europe, have used monitoring of portal pressures and hepatic venous pressure gradient through transjugular catheterization in clinical practice; however, the invasive nature of this technique has limited its application in most centers around the world. If further studies corroborate the safety and reliability of EUS-guided portal pressure measurement, this technique could also be part of the evaluation during EUS-guided liver biopsy and EGD for variceal screening/surveillance.

Advanced endoscopic interventions have also extended into bariatric procedures, offering truly minimally invasive options, such as endoscopic sleeve gastroplasty and endoscopic duodenal mucosal resurfacing, for the management of obesity and related comorbid conditions. The obesity epidemic has propelled metabolic-associated fatty liver disease to be one of the leading causes of chronic liver disease in Western countries. Although traditional bariatric surgical interventions have proven to improve hepatic steatosis, steatohepatitis, metabolic parameters and to diminish fibrosis, patients with chronic liver disease are frequently considered at high risk for surgical complications, thus the need for less invasive alternatives. However, what is most intriguing about endoscopic bariatric interventions is not only their minimally invasive nature and proven efficacy in achieving weight loss but also their positive impact on metabolic derangements, such as insulin resistance and improvements in hepatic fibrosis.

On behalf of all the contributors, I sincerely hope that this special issue of the *Clinics in Liver Disease* stimulates further discussion, collaboration, and research between hepatologists and advanced endoscopists to continue improving the care of patients with chronic liver diseases.

Andres F. Carrion, MD
Division of Digestive Health and Liver Diseases
University of Miami Miller School of Medicine
1120 Northwest 14th Street, Suite 1189
Miami, FL 33136, USA

E-mail address:
acarrion@med.miami.edu

Management of Thrombocytopenia and Coagulopathy in Patients with Chronic Liver Disease Undergoing Therapeutic Endoscopic Interventions

Jay Luther, MD[a,b,c], Lawrence S. Friedman, MD[b,c,d,e],*

KEYWORDS

- Cirrhosis • Colonoscopy • Esophagogastroduodenoscopy
- Endoscopic variceal ligation • Fibrinogen • Fresh frozen plasma • Platelets
- Thrombopoietin

KEY POINTS

- Patients with advanced liver disease have alterations in both anticoagulant and procoagulant factors.
- Available tests of hemostasis all have major limitations in assessing bleeding risk in patients with liver disease.
- In patients with cirrhosis, additional factors that affect bleeding risk include clinically significant portal hypertension, infection, and kidney disease.
- Endoscopic procedures may be classified as low risk or high risk with regard to bleeding.
- Fresh frozen plasma should not be administered to patients with cirrhosis before endoscopic procedures. In selected cases platelet transfusions, a thrombopoietin agonist, or supplementation of fibrinogen, may be considered.

The management of coagulopathy in patients with advanced liver disease undergoing therapeutic endoscopic procedures is complex. Improvements in the understanding of hemostasis at a physiologic level have highlighted the inaccuracy of currently

[a] MGH Alcohol Liver Center, Boston, MA, USA; [b] Division of Gastroenterology, Department of Medicine, Massachusetts General Hospital, Blake 4, 55 Fruit Street, Boston, MA 02114, USA; [c] Department of Medicine, Harvard Medical School, Boston, MA, USA; [d] Department of Medicine, Newton-Wellesley Hospital, Newton, MA, USA; [e] Department of Medicine, Tufts University School of Medicine, Boston, MA, USA
* Corresponding author. Newton-Wellesley Hospital, 2014 Washington Street, Newton, MA 02462.
E-mail address: lfriedman@partners.org

Clin Liver Dis 26 (2022) 1–12
https://doi.org/10.1016/j.cld.2021.08.002
1089-3261/22/© 2021 Elsevier Inc. All rights reserved.

liver.theclinics.com

available clinical tests, such as the platelet count and prothrombin time, in estimating hemostasis in patients with cirrhosis. Furthermore, with identification of novel factors that contribute to bleeding risk in patients with cirrhosis, there is a dearth of clinical trial data that account for all potentially relevant factors and that examine interventions to reduce bleeding risk. For these reasons, precise recommendations regarding transfusion strategies based on hemostatic test results in patients with cirrhosis are impractical.

THE BIOLOGY OF HEMOSTASIS IN PATIENTS WITH CIRRHOSIS

Regulation of hemostasis in patients with cirrhosis is complex. Despite more than 60 years of research on this topic, the understanding of coagulation in patients with cirrhosis remains imperfect. Over this time period, there have been multiple shifts in the perception of bleeding risk. Initially, patients with cirrhosis were thought to exhibit a propensity for bleeding. It had been well established that the hepatocyte is the primary cell responsible for production of coagulation factors, so it followed that patients with chronic liver disease would be expected to have an increased risk of bleeding. In fact, multiple mechanistic studies supported this hypothesis. First, impaired hepatocyte function leads to a reduction in the synthesis of certain procoagulant factors, such as fibrinogen, thrombin, and factors V, VII, IX, X, and XI. Second, hepatocytes are critical for posttranslational modifications of coagulation factors, a process that is impaired when hepatocyte function is reduced. Third, liver disease is associated with decreased levels of alpha-1 antitrypsin and thrombin-activatable fibrinolysis inhibitor, along with elevated levels of fibrin degradation products, and may promote hyperfibrinolysis.[1,2] Fourth, patients with cirrhosis have a decrease in the production of thrombopoietin (TPO) and increased splenic sequestration of platelets, and older data suggested that platelet aggregation and adhesion are impaired in this population.[3–6] Finally, many coagulation factors are dependent on vitamin K, levels of which may be decreased in patients with liver disease. Taken together, multiple hemostatic alterations that drive a propensity to bleeding are common in persons with liver disease and have led to the perception that these patients are prone to bleeding.

Nevertheless, the understanding of the dynamic changes in hemostasis has evolved over time. In contrast to previous work, subsequent research also identified deficiencies in hepatocyte-dependent production of fibrinolytic factors and inhibitors of coagulation in patients with cirrhosis. Many of these abnormalities directly counteract the previously identified probleeding pathways. Furthermore, impaired hepatocyte function limits production of proteins C and S and antithrombin, thereby promoting clot formation. Patients with chronic liver disease also have increased serum levels of plasminogen activator inhibitor and reduced serum levels of plasminogen, ultimately decreasing fibrinolysis. Similarly, patients with cirrhosis exhibit elevated levels of von Willebrand factor (VWF), likely because of reduced levels of VWF-cleaving protease (ADAMTS13), which counteracts the dysfunction in platelet aggregation and adhesion. As opposed to the other procoagulant factors, levels of factor VIII, which is produced by hepatic sinusoidal cells and not hepatocytes, may be increased in patients with cirrhosis.[7,8] These data support clinical studies suggesting that patients with cirrhosis may in fact have a propensity to clotting, particularly a higher tendency to splanchnic thrombosis, compared with patients without cirrhosis.[9,10]

Traditionally, hepatocytes were thought to be the main drivers of coagulation status in patients with liver disease, but it is becoming evident that other cell types are critical as well. For example, activated neutrophils, which have numerous roles in liver disease, are capable of producing neutrophil extracellular traps, which in turn have the capability to promote the progression of hypercoagulability.[11,12] Erythrocytes can also influence coagulation through their effects on endothelial adherence, platelet function, and the levels of coagulant factors.[13] Endothelial cells, in addition to their role in VWF production, may also have important effects on coagulation, especially in patients with cirrhosis.[14] Moreover, the function of all these cell types is influenced by infection, systemic inflammation, medications, and kidney disease.[15] These observations reinforce the complexity of hemostasis in patients with liver disease, because many patients with liver disease also experience systemic complications. With the continued identification of novel cellular contributors to hemostasis, coupled with a better understanding of the dynamic relation between procoagulant and anticoagulant pathways, we may ultimately be better able to predict the true risk of bleeding and thrombosis in patients with cirrhosis.

TESTS TO MEASURE COAGULATION STATUS IN PATIENTS WITH CIRRHOSIS

Improved understanding of the complexities of coagulation in patients with cirrhosis makes currently available clinical tests to estimate bleeding risk unreliable (**Table 1**). All currently used tests do not account for the dynamic changes that occur in both the procoagulant and the anticoagulant pathways. For example, thrombocytopenia (defined as a platelet count <50,000/mm^3) has traditionally been associated with an increased bleeding risk. For reasons discussed earlier, patients with cirrhosis commonly have platelet counts less than this threshold. However, the absolute platelet count does not account for other dynamic procoagulant changes that occur in patients with cirrhosis or the potential enhancement of platelet function via increased synthesis of VWF.[7] Furthermore, patients with preserved renal function may exhibit improved platelet aggregation and secretion, independent of VWF, compared with patients without concurrent renal disease.[15] In line with these data, multiple clinical studies have shown no association between the preprocedural platelet count and bleeding risk, independent of portal hypertension, in patients with cirrhosis.[16,17] The bleeding time is no longer commonly used in clinical practice, because it also is not a reliable measure of coagulopathy or bleeding risk in patients with cirrhosis.

Table 1
Limitations to currently available hemostatic tests in patients with cirrhosis

Test	Limitations
Platelet count	Does not account for enhancement in platelet function, aggregation, and secretion
Bleeding time	Outdated (not used clinically); use in past was based solely on platelet function without an assessment of other hemostatic changes
PT (INR), PTT	Do not account for pathway-independent changes in coagulation; no data to support increased bleeding risk in patients with prolonged values
Serum fibrinogen level	Clinical data to support its use are confounded by other clinical factors (such as critical illness)
Global assessments of hemostasis (eg, thromboelastography)	Unable to detect platelet dysfunction and assess the effects of VWF; not sensitive to the activity of proteins C and S and antithrombin

Abbreviations: INR, international normalized ratio; PT, prothrombin time PTT, partial thromboplastin time; VWF, von Willebrand factor.

Patients with cirrhosis commonly present with a prolongation of the prothrombin time and an increase in the international normalized ratio (INR) and partial thromboplastin time (PTT) as a result of impaired synthesis of procoagulant factors. Although these abnormalities in isolation might predict bleeding risk, they do not account for many of the procoagulant changes that occur in parallel. For this reason, although an elevation in the INR may signify hepatic dysfunction, it does not provide an accurate estimate of bleeding risk in patients with cirrhosis. Accordingly, multiple clinical studies have demonstrated the lack of an increase in bleeding risk when the INR is elevated in patients with liver disease undergoing procedures such as paracentesis or endoscopic variceal ligation (EVL).[18,19] Accordingly, traditionally set thresholds for an INR of 1.5, or even 2.0 in some cases, are not associated with bleeding risk.[20] For this reason, it is generally thought that the INR provides little indication of the bleeding tendency in patients with cirrhosis. Similarly, elevated PTT values are not associated with an increased risk of bleeding in patients with cirrhosis and therefore are not an indication for targeted therapy to correct these values.

Serum levels of fibrinogen may offer insight into bleeding risk. Fibrinogen levels less than 100 mg/dL have been associated with bleeding in patients with cirrhosis, thereby suggesting that at these low levels of fibrinogen, the procoagulant changes that occur simultaneously may not be able to fully compensate for the low fibrinogen levels.[21,22] Most patients with low levels of fibrinogen in these clinical studies, however, were critically ill, thereby raising the possibility that a low fibrinogen level may serve as a proxy for critical illness, which may in fact be driving the bleeding tendency. Therefore, although low fibrinogen levels may be associated with bleeding risk, it is not clear that the risk is directly related to reduced fibrinogen levels.

GLOBAL ASSESSMENTS OF HEMOSTASIS IN PATIENTS WITH CIRRHOSIS

Given the inherent deficiencies in the commonly used clinical tests to estimate bleeding risk in patients with cirrhosis, there is interest in clinically accurate and feasible tests that account for the dynamic and global changes in hemostasis. Perhaps most promising is the use of viscoelastic testing, in particular, thromboelastography (TEG) and rotational thromboelastometry (ROTEM), to estimate bleeding risk. TEG, for example, uses a probe that assesses changes in viscosity (measured as clot signal units) over time that occur within a blood sample that is positionally rotated, thereby stimulating solid clot formation. Using mathematical interpretation of changes in viscosity over time, TEG allows measurements of the time to clot formation, speed of clot formation, and clot strength and thus an overall assessment of coagulability. Although TEG and related tests were developed decades ago, they have only been well studied recently in patients with cirrhosis. TEG has been studied as (1) a measure of coagulopathy before invasive procedures; (2) a guide to transfusion in patients experiencing gastrointestinal bleeding or undergoing liver transplantation; and (3) an assessment of bleeding risk in patients with an acute decompensation of liver disease.[23] A randomized, controlled trial examining TEG-guided blood product use before invasive procedures in patients with cirrhosis found that TEG-guided therapy led to a reduction in blood product use compared with an approach guided by the INR and platelet count, without leading to an increased risk in bleeding.[24] Although these results are promising, certain limitations, such as the inability of TEG to detect platelet dysfunction and assess the effects of VWF, may lead to an underestimation of coagulation in some patients.[25] Furthermore, TEG is not sensitive to the activity of proteins C and S, as well as antithrombin. For these reasons, further clinical studies examining the accuracy and clinical utility of TEG (and ROTEM) are needed.

Plasma-based thrombin generation tests (TGTs) measure the overall tendency to form thrombin[26] and, when supplemented with thrombomodulin or protein C activators, may offer an accurate assessment of coagulation balance. However, these tests are technically cumbersome, thereby limiting their use in clinical practice. Development of operator friendly and cost-efficient TGTs is needed before more widespread use in clinical practice.[27]

PATIENT-RELATED FACTORS THAT INFLUENCE BLEEDING RISK IN PATIENTS WITH CIRRHOSIS

Emerging data have identified several patient-related factors that are critical in determining bleeding risk in patients with cirrhosis (**Box 1**). For example, patients with clinically significant portal hypertension are at increased risk of bleeding compared with those with well-compensated disease.[28] Patients with an acute decompensation of liver disease are also more likely to have bleeding complications during invasive procedures, independent of INR and platelet count.[29] These data support the notion that more advanced liver disease is likely to be associated with an increased risk of bleeding.

In addition to liver-specific factors, patients with certain systemic factors may exhibit an increased risk of bleeding. Perhaps the most well-studied systemic risk factor in patients with cirrhosis is the presence of kidney disease. One study found that patients who experienced bleeding following EVL had a significantly higher serum creatinine level than those who did not bleed after the procedure (2.2 mg/dL for bleeders vs 1.0 mg/dL for nonbleeders; $P = .001$). This difference was independent of the platelet count and INR.[30] In addition, patients taking antiplatelet or anticoagulant medications may also exhibit an increased risk of bleeding. Although this makes intuitive sense, it is important to note that the association between anticoagulant use and bleeding in patients with cirrhosis is not straightforward, with some studies suggesting no relationship.[31] This finding, coupled with a potential benefit in the overall mortality of anticoagulation in patients with cirrhosis,[32] highlights the need for further research on this topic.

BLEEDING RISK OF ENDOSCOPIC PROCEDURES

Although patient-related factors are critical in determining the potential for bleeding in a patient with cirrhosis undergoing an endoscopic procedure, it is important to recognize that various endoscopic procedures have different risks of associated bleeding (**Box 2**). In general, any endoscopic procedure that entails an intervention is more

---

Box 1
Clinical factors associated with bleeding risk in patients with cirrhosis undergoing endoscopic procedures

Severity of liver disease
   Presence of portal hypertension
   Child-Pugh class

Medical comorbidities
   Renal disease
   Medications (eg, anticoagulants)

Endoscopic procedure
   Low vs high risk (see **Box 2**)

Box 2
Classification of endoscopic procedures commonly performed in patients with cirrhosis based on bleeding risk

Low risk (<1.5%)
  EGD
  EGD with argon plasma coagulation
  Colonoscopy
  Colonoscopy with mucosal biopsies
  Colonoscopy with removal of polyps <1 cm in size
  ERCP without sphincterotomy
  EUS without fine needle aspiration/biopsy

High risk (≥1.5%)
  EGD with EVL
  Colonoscopy with removal of polyps ≥1 cm in size
  ERCP with sphincterotomy
  EUS with fine needle aspiration/biopsy

Abbreviations: EGD, esophagogastroduodenoscopy; ERCP, endoscopic retrograde cholangio-pancreatography; EUS, endoscopic ultrasonography; EVL, endoscopic variceal ligation.

---

likely to cause bleeding than a procedure without an intervention. Endoscopic procedures can be classified as those associated with a low risk of bleeding (<1.5%) and those associated with a high risk of bleeding (≥1.5%). Low-risk procedures commonly performed in patients with cirrhosis include esophagogastroduodenoscopy (EGD), EGD with argon plasma coagulation therapy, colonoscopy with mucosal biopsies or removal of polyps less than 1 cm in diameter, and endoscopic retrograde cholangio-pancreatography (ERCP) without sphincterotomy. Limited data on bleeding risk following polypectomy in patients with cirrhosis support a low risk of bleeding (0.3%), comparable to rates in patients without liver disease.[33] Advanced liver disease, defined by the presence of ascites and/or esophageal varices, and cold-snare polypectomy were identified as potential predictors of bleeding risk. Characteristics of the polyp (size, morphology, and histology) were not associated with the risk of bleeding. Commonly performed high-risk procedures in patients with cirrhosis include EGD with EVL, colonoscopy with large polyp (≥1 cm) removal, and ERCP with sphincterotomy.[34] The most recent data suggest a bleeding risk of approximately 5% in patients with cirrhosis undergoing prophylactic EVL, with perhaps a slightly higher risk in those patients with advanced liver disease and large varices.[35] Understanding the risks of various endoscopic procedures helps determine preendoscopy management strategies to minimize the risk of bleeding.

EFFICACY OF THRESHOLD-BASED TRANSFUSION STRATEGIES IN PATIENTS WITH CIRRHOSIS
Thrombocytopenia

The notion that a low platelet count would increase the bleeding risk, and that correction of a low platelet count to a certain threshold would attenuate the bleeding risk, seems logical. However, this is likely not the case in patients with cirrhosis, for multiple reasons. First, as noted previously, the absolute platelet count may not correlate with the bleeding risk in patients undergoing endoscopic procedures. Second, data have highlighted the inability of platelet transfusions to improve global tests of hemostasis in patients with cirrhosis, even in those with baseline severe thrombocytopenia.[36] Third, there is a paucity of data examining the efficacy of platelet transfusions on procedural bleeding risk in patients with cirrhosis. In fact, some data suggest that patients with liver disease who receive platelet transfusions may paradoxically be at an increased risk of bleeding.[37] Finally, platelet transfusions are not risk-free and have been associated with the development of transfusion-related lung injury syndromes. For these reasons, data are lacking to support platelet transfusions based solely on the platelet count in patients with cirrhosis undergoing endoscopic procedures.

Medical therapies to elevate the platelet count have been developed as an alternative to platelet transfusions. These medications, some of which, including avatrombopag and lusutrombopag, have recently been approved by the Food and Drug Administration, leverage the known biology of platelet physiology to stimulate bone marrow production of platelets through TPO receptor agonism, increase the platelet count, and reduce the need for platelet transfusions in patients with cirrhosis.[38] However, use of these medications has not been demonstrated to reduce bleeding risk in patients with cirrhosis undergoing endoscopic procedures. Furthermore, concerns regarding the potential for an increased risk of thrombotic events have been raised in patients receiving these medications.[39] It is also important to note that these medications must be administered for multiple days before a procedure in order to raise the platelet count, and their effects can last upwards of 2 weeks. Taken together, data are lacking to support empiric medical therapy to elevate the platelet count in patients with cirrhosis.

Factor Deficiencies

Patients with cirrhosis commonly exhibit an elevated INR; however, as noted previously, an elevated INR is unlikely to provide meaningful insight into the overall coagulation status of patients with cirrhosis. It is not surprising, therefore, that targeting a particular INR threshold before endoscopy has not been shown to offer benefit in reducing the bleeding risk in patients with cirrhosis. First, the ability of an elevated INR to independently predict bleeding risk in a patient with cirrhosis is poor.[28] Second, clinical data are lacking to support the use of fresh frozen plasma (FFP) transfusions in patients with cirrhosis to reduce the bleeding risk before endoscopy. A multicenter, retrospective study examining the association between FFP transfusions and mortality in patients with cirrhosis who presented with acute variceal hemorrhage found an almost 10-fold increased risk of mortality and a 3-fold increased risk of persistent bleeding in patients who received FFP transfusions compared with those who did not receive FFP transfusions, independent of the severity of the underlying liver disease and the presence of active bleeding on index examination.[40] Therefore, the routine use of FFP to correct an elevated INR in patients with cirrhosis cannot be recommended.

Fibrinogen

Low serum fibrinogen levels can be found in patients with cirrhosis, especially those who are critically ill.[41] Unfortunately, clinically available tests that estimate hyperfibrinolysis are lacking. Furthermore, there are insufficient clinical trial data on the effect of infusions of fibrinogen-rich products, such as cryoprecipitate, on procedural bleeding risk in patients with cirrhosis. Randomized clinical trials examining the effect of tranexamic acid on bleeding risk and mortality rates in patients presenting with acute gastrointestinal bleeding showed no benefit and, in fact, identified an increased risk of thrombosis associated with administration of tranexamic acid in patients with cirrhosis.[42] For these reasons, a transfusion strategy based solely on fibrinogen levels in patients with cirrhosis undergoing endoscopic procedures cannot be recommended.

Hemoglobin

Randomized, clinical trial data have demonstrated a mortality benefit for transfusion of packed red blood cells to a hemoglobin level of 7 g/dL, compared with 9 g/dL, in patients with cirrhosis presenting with upper gastrointestinal bleeding.[43] Although all patients with cirrhosis benefited from a more restrictive approach to red blood cell transfusions, the benefit was most pronounced in patients with Child-Pugh class A or B cirrhosis. A survival advantage was seen in patients presenting with variceal and peptic ulcer bleeding, reinforcing the benefit of restricting packed red blood cell transfusions to those patients with cirrhosis who present with a hemoglobin of less than 7 g/dL.

RECOMMENDATIONS OF PROFESSIONAL SOCIETIES

Given the complexity of this topic, there is variability in the recommendations made by the major gastrointestinal and hepatology societies with regard to managing patients with cirrhosis before endoscopy. A 2020 guidance put forth by the American Association for the Study of Liver Diseases was the first to suggest a threshold-based transfusion strategy before endoscopy in patients with cirrhosis.[28] The guidance rejects taking measures aimed at reducing the INR before any procedures. It also stresses the importance of individualizing the approach to each patient, especially when it comes to managing thrombocytopenia and low fibrinogen levels. For example, the guidance suggests consideration of fibrinogen transfusions aiming for plasma fibrinogen levels greater than 100 mg/dL before high-risk procedures while also acknowledging that data to support this recommendation are lacking. The guidance statement published by the American College of Gastroenterology (ACG) in 2020 suggests against FFP administration before procedures.[44] Although also not recommending platelet transfusions across the board in patients with cirrhosis who have a platelet count less than 50,000/mm^3, the ACG guidance does suggest transfusions or administration of TPO agonists for patients with concurrent renal disease or those undergoing high-risk endoscopic procedures.[44] A guidance statement from the American Gastroenterological Association published in 2019 supports the use of platelet transfusions or TPO agonists to achieve a platelet count of at least 50,000/mm^3 in patients undergoing high-risk endoscopic procedures.[45] The inconsistency in recommendations made by these societies highlights the controversies associated with this topic, the importance of individualizing the clinical decision in each patient, and the need for further research.

SUMMARY

The understanding of hemostasis in patients with cirrhosis is evolving. For this reason, the evaluation of a patient with advanced liver disease before endoscopy requires careful attention to clinical circumstance. As previously discussed, bleeding risk in patients with cirrhosis depends on multiple factors, including the severity of liver disease, presence of coexisting systemic diseases known to accentuate bleeding risk, presence of portal hypertension, and type of procedure being performed. Any approach to the management of patients that attempts to reduce the bleeding risk in patients with advanced liver disease before endoscopy should address these factors. The authors agree with the recommendation of the professional societies that in no clinical scenario should FFP be administered to lower the INR before endoscopy, given the lack of efficacy and potential complications associated with administration of FFP, including transfusion-related syndromes and circulatory overload.

Table 2
Suggested management of thrombocytopenia and coagulopathy in patients with advanced liver disease undergoing endoscopic procedures[a]

| | Bleeding Risk of Endoscopic Procedure | |
	Low	High
Patient characteristics	Nonadvanced liver disease No renal disease No anticoagulation	Advanced liver disease Renal disease On anticoagulation
Strategy	No transfusions	Transfusion to target[b]: Platelets >50,000/mm³ Fibrinogen >100 mg/dL

[a] Based on the bleeding risk (low or high) of the endoscopic procedure.
[b] Thrombopoietin agonist in patients undergoing endoscopic variceal ligation.

The authors' suggested approach begins with identifying the bleeding risk of the endoscopic procedure being performed (**Table 2**). In patients undergoing endoscopic procedures with a low bleeding risk, such as routine EGD or colonoscopy with the potential for removal of small (<1 cm) polyps, there is likely no benefit to transfusions of platelets, regardless of the patient's absolute platelet count. For patients undergoing high-risk endoscopic procedures, more clinical information is needed before making management decisions. The presence of coexisting renal disease, systemic infection, or use of antithrombotic medications may increase a patient's bleeding risk independent of liver disease, and in these situations, achieving a platelet count greater than 50,000/mm³ should be considered. Although EGD with EVL is classified as a high-risk bleeding procedure, the bleeding associated with this procedure is usually delayed until 5 to 10 days after the procedure. Accordingly, the administration of platelets is unlikely to have a sustained benefit in these patients.[46] Administration of a TPO agonist, however, provides more sustained elevations in the platelet count and should be considered in this clinical setting, if time permits. Finally, in any patient with known active bleeding undergoing endoscopy, platelet transfusions to maintain a platelet count greater than 50,000/mm³ and supplementation of fibrinogen to maintain a level greater than 100 mg/dL should be considered. In the future, it is hoped that global tests of hemostasis, such as TEG, will be further validated and provide an objective marker to guide clinicians when faced with this clinical challenge. Randomized clinical trial data are needed to definitively address the benefits and risks of threshold-based transfusion strategies.

CLINICS CARE POINTS

- Traditional clinical markers of hemostasis (platelets, PTT, INR) are not reliable in patients with cirrhosis.
- Aim for a target hemoglobin level of >7 g/dL in patients with cirrhosis and bleeding.
- There is no threshold value of INR that is needed prior to performing endoscopy.
- Consider transfusion of platelets to a target of 50,000/mm³ in high-risk patients undergoing high-risk endoscopic procedures.

DISCLOSURE

J. Luther: None. L.S. Friedman: None.

REFERENCES

1. Van Thiel DH, George M, Fareed J. Low levels of thrombin activatable fibrinolysis inhibitor (TAFI) in patients with chronic liver disease. Thromb Haemost 2001; 85(4):667–70.
2. Bedreli S, Sowa JP, Malek S, et al. Rotational thromboelastometry can detect factor XIII deficiency and bleeding diathesis in patients with cirrhosis. Liver Int 2017; 37(4):562–8.
3. Finkbiner RB, McGovern JJ, Goldstein R, et al. Coagulation defects in liver disease and response to transfusion during surgery. Am J Med 1959;26(2):199–213.
4. Roberts HR, Cederbaum AI. The liver and blood coagulation: physiology and pathology. Gastroenterology 1972;63(2):297–320.
5. Devenyi P, Robinson GM, Kapur BM, et al. High-density lipoprotein cholesterol in male alcoholics with and without severe liver disease. Am J Med 1981;71(4): 589–94.
6. Hugenholtz GGC, Porte RJ, Lisman T. The platelet and platelet function testing in liver disease. Clin Liver Dis 2009;13(1):11–20.
7. Lisman T, Bongers TN, Adelmeijer J, et al. Elevated levels of von Willebrand factor in cirrhosis support platelet adhesion despite reduced functional capacity. Hepatology 2006;44(1):53–61.
8. Gómez MR, García ES, Lacomba DL, et al. Antiphospholipid antibodies are related to portal vein thrombosis in patients with liver cirrhosis. J Clin Gastroenterol 2000;31(3):237–40.
9. Amitrano L, Guardascione MA, Ames PRJ. Coagulation abnormalities in cirrhotic patients with portal vein thrombosis. Clin Lab 2007;53(9–12):583–9.
10. Zermatten MG, Fraga M, Moradpour D, et al. Hemostatic alterations in patients with cirrhosis: from primary hemostasis to fibrinolysis. Hepatology 2020;71(6): 2135–48.
11. Wolach O, Sellar RS, Martinod K, et al. Increased neutrophil extracellular trap formation promotes thrombosis in myeloproliferative neoplasms. Sci Transl Med 2018;10(436):8292.
12. Martinod K, Wagner DD. Thrombosis: tangled up in NETs. Blood 2014;123(18): 2768–76.
13. Weisel JW, Litvinov RI. Red blood cells: the forgotten player in hemostasis and thrombosis. J Thromb Haemost 2019;17(2):271–82.
14. Shalaby S, Simioni P, Campello E, et al. Endothelial damage of the portal vein is associated with heparin-like effect in advanced stages of cirrhosis. Thromb Haemost 2020;120(8):1173–81.
15. Zanetto A, Rinder HM, Campello E, et al. Acute kidney injury in decompensated cirrhosis is associated with both hypo-coagulable and hyper-coagulable features. Hepatology 2020;72(4):1327–40.
16. Basili S, Raparelli V, Napoleone L, et al. Platelet count does not predict bleeding in cirrhotic patients: results from the PRO-LIVER Study. Am J Gastroenterol 2018; 113(3):368–75.
17. Napolitano G, Iacobellis A, Merla A, et al. Bleeding after invasive procedures is rare and unpredicted by platelet counts in cirrhotic patients with thrombocytopenia. Eur J Intern Med 2017;38:79–82.
18. Grabau CM, Crago SF, Hoff LK, et al. Performance standards for therapeutic abdominal paracentesis. Hepatology 2004;40(2):484–8.

19. Vieira da Rocha EC, D'Amico EA, Caldwell SH, et al. A prospective study of conventional and expanded coagulation indices in predicting ulcer bleeding after variceal band ligation. Clin Gastroenterol Hepatol 2009;7(9):988–93.
20. Andriulli A, Tripodi A, Angeli P, et al. Hemostatic balance in patients with liver cirrhosis: report of a consensus conference. Dig Liver Dis 2016;48(5):455–67.
21. Drolz A, Horvatits T, Roedl K, et al. Coagulation parameters and major bleeding in critically ill patients with cirrhosis. Hepatology 2016;64(2):556–68.
22. Giannini EG, Giambruno E, Brunacci M, et al. Low fibrinogen levels are associated with bleeding after varices ligation in thrombocytopenic cirrhotic patients. Ann Hepatol 2018;17(5):830–5.
23. Shenoy A, Intagliata NM. Thromboelastography and utility in hepatology practice. Clin Liver Dis 2020;16(4):149–52.
24. De Pietri L, Bianchini M, Montalti R, et al. Thrombelastography-guided blood product use before invasive procedures in cirrhosis with severe coagulopathy: a randomized, controlled trial. Hepatology 2016;63(2):566–73.
25. Schepis F, Turco L, Bianchini M, et al. Prevention and management of bleeding risk related to invasive procedures in cirrhosis. Semin Liver Dis 2018;38(3):215–29.
26. Castoldi E, Rosing J. Thrombin generation tests. Thromb Res 2011;127(SUPPL. 3):S21–5.
27. Talon L, Sinegre T, Lecompte T, et al. Hypercoagulability (thrombin generation) in patients with cirrhosis is detected with ST-Genesia. J Thromb Haemost 2020;18(9):2177–90.
28. Northup PG, Garcia-Pagan JC, Garcia-Tsao G, et al. Vascular liver disorders, portal vein thrombosis, and procedural bleeding in patients with liver disease: 2020 Practice Guidance by the American Association for the Study of Liver Diseases. Hepatology 2021;73(1):366–413.
29. Lin S, Wang M, Zhu Y, et al. Hemorrhagic complications following abdominal paracentesis in acute on chronic liver failure a propensity score analysis. Medicine (Baltimore) 2015;94(49):e2225.
30. Bianchini M, Cavani G, Bonaccorso A, et al. Low molecular weight heparin does not increase bleeding and mortality post-endoscopic variceal band ligation in cirrhotic patients. Liver Int 2018;38(7):1253–62.
31. Cerini F, Gonzalez JM, Torres F, et al. Impact of anticoagulation on upper-gastrointestinal bleeding in cirrhosis. A retrospective multicenter study. Hepatology 2015;62(2):575–83.
32. Villa E, Cammà C, Marietta M, et al. Enoxaparin prevents portal vein thrombosis and liver decompensation in patients with advanced cirrhosis. Gastroenterology 2012;143(5):1253–60.
33. Huang R, Perumpail R, Thosani N, et al. Colonoscopy with polypectomy is associated with a low rate of complications in patients with cirrhosis. Endosc Int Open 2016;04(09):E947–52.
34. Acosta RD, Abraham NS, Chandrasekhara V, et al. The management of antithrombotic agents for patients undergoing GI endoscopy. Gastrointest Endosc 2016;83(1):3–16.
35. Drolz A, Schramm C, Seiz O, et al. Risk factors associated with bleeding after prophylactic endoscopic variceal ligation in cirrhosis. Endoscopy 2021;53(3):226–34.
36. Tripodi A, Primignani M, Chantarangkul V, et al. Global hemostasis tests in patients with cirrhosis before and after prophylactic platelet transfusion. Liver Int 2013;33(3):362–7.

37. Giannini EG, Greco A, Marenco S, et al. Incidence of bleeding following invasive procedures in patients with thrombocytopenia and advanced liver disease. Clin Gastroenterol Hepatol 2010;8(10):899–902.
38. Terrault N, Chen YC, Izumi N, et al. Avatrombopag before procedures reduces need for platelet transfusion in patients with chronic liver disease and thrombocytopenia. Gastroenterology 2018;155(3):705–18.
39. Afdhal NH, Giannini EG, Tayyab G, et al. Eltrombopag before procedures in patients with cirrhosis and thrombocytopenia. N Engl J Med 2012;367(8):716–24.
40. Mohanty A, Kapuria D, Canakis A, et al. Fresh frozen plasma transfusion in acute variceal haemorrhage: results from a multicentre cohort study. Liver Int 2021; 40(8):1901–8.
41. Tripodi A, Primignani M, Chantarangkul V, et al. An imbalance of pro- vs anticoagulation factors in plasma from patients with cirrhosis. Gastroenterology 2009;137(6):2105–11.
42. HALT-IT Trial Collaborators. Effects of a high-dose 24-h infusion of tranexamic acid on death and thromboembolic events in patients with acute gastrointestinal bleeding (HALT-IT): an international randomised, double-blind, placebo-controlled trial. Lancet 2020;395(10241):1927–36.
43. Villanueva C, Colomo A, Bosch A, et al. Transfusion strategies for acute upper gastrointestinal bleeding. N Engl J Med 2013;368(1):11–21.
44. Simonetto DA, Singal AK, Garcia-Tsao G, et al. ACG clinical guideline: disorders of the hepatic and mesenteric circulation. Am J Gastroenterol 2020;115(1):18–40.
45. O'Leary JG, Greenberg CS, Patton HM, et al. AGA clinical practice update: coagulation in cirrhosis. Gastroenterology 2019;157(1):34–43.
46. Blasi A, Cardenas A. Invasive procedures in patients with cirrhosis: a clinical approach based on current evidence. Clin Liver Dis 2021;25(2):461–70.

Polypectomy, Endoscopic Mucosal Resection, and Endoscopic Submucosal Dissection in the Cirrhotic Population

Ahmad Nakshabandi, MD[a], Manasi Rungta, BS[b],
Mohamed O. Othman, MD[b,c],*

KEYWORDS

- EMR • ESD • Cirrhosis • Endoscopy • Advanced endoscopy • Adverse events
- Bleeding • Perforation

KEY POINTS

- Adverse events with endoscopic mucosal resection and dissection are higher in the cirrhotic population.
- Endoscopic submucosal dissection (ESD) in cirrhotic patients is associated with frequent intraprocedural bleeding.
- ESD for esophageal and rectal lesions in the presence of varices is possible but requires significant experience to separate the lesion from the underlying varices in the submucosa with meticulous dissection.

INTRODUCTION

Endoscopic mucosal resection (EMR) and endoscopic submucosal dissection (ESD) are endoscopic techniques of a minimally invasive nature that have been developed for the removal of benign and early malignant lesions in the mucosal layer as well as the submucosal layer. In the mid-1950s, EMR technique was first introduced as a method whereby a saline solution was injected into the submucosal space under the lesion, creating a safety cushion whereby the lesion could then be removed in a single resection or by piecemeal fashion.[1] EMR techniques evolved over time and now include standard EMR, underwater EMR, and snare tip soft coagulation EMR.[2,3]

[a] Department of Gastroenterology & Hepatology, MedStar Georgetown University Hospital, 3800 Reservoir Rd NW, Washington, DC 20007, USA; [b] Gastroenterology and Hepatology Section, Baylor College of Medicine, 7200 Cambridge Street, 8th Floor, Suite 8B, Houston, TX 77030, USA; [c] Gastroenterology Section, BSLMC, Baylor College of Medicine, 7200 Cambridge Street, 8th Floor, Suite 8B, Houston, TX 77030, USA
* Corresponding author.
E-mail address: Mohamed.othman@bcm.edu

Clin Liver Dis 26 (2022) 13–19
https://doi.org/10.1016/j.cld.2021.09.001
1089-3261/22/© 2021 Elsevier Inc. All rights reserved.

In contrast, ESD techniques allow en bloc resection of the lesion after careful dissection of the submucosal space. This technique was first described in 1988 as an alternative to surgery for the treatment of early gastric neoplasia.[4] The principles of ESD have since developed into more therapeutic options for other pathologies of the gastrointestinal tract including resections of early esophageal cancer and complex colonic polyps.

These minimally invasive endoluminal resection techniques have yielded positive outcomes for numerous advanced premalignant and early low-grade malignant lesions. However, a continued topic of interest is the potential adverse outcomes related to these procedures, including bleeding and perforation in average-risk patients and more so in cirrhotic populations. In this review, we will focus on the outcomes of EMR and ESD in cirrhotic patients with a focus on the risk of bleeding and perforation.

INDICATIONS FOR ENDOSCOPIC RESECTION

Both EMR and ESD procedures may be carried out in the upper and lower gastrointestinal tract. Lesions amenable to EMR in the upper gastrointestinal tract include those less than 20 mm in size with low risk of submucosal invasion. Lesions in the upper gastrointestinal tract demonstrate that submucosal invasion or intramucosal carcinoma should be considered for ESD, including lesions that previously underwent EMR which demonstrate positive margin or previous incomplete resection. The limitation in the size and depth of invasion underscore the advantages of ESD over EMR. En bloc resection of any lesion size can be performed by ESD, which also yields precise pathology review of lateral, and deep margins.[5,6]

Colorectal lesions can undergo EMR to resect large colonic polyps by piecemeal technique, whereas the ESD technique is typically reserved for colorectal lesions with features suggestive of high-grade dysplasia or early carcinoma, particularly nongranular lateral spreading tumors.[7] Colorectal lesions resected via EMR or ESD are associated with lower mortality in comparison to surgical resections. In a prospective trial of 1050 patients with colorectal lesions treated by EMR, the actual 30-day mortality rate was 0% than the predicated 5% mortality rate typically seen in surgical resections.[8]

OUTCOMES OF ENDOSCOPIC RESECTION TECHNIQUES

A meta-analysis evaluated curative and recurrence rates following ESD versus EMR procedures on early esophageal adenocarcinoma which demonstrated curative resection rates of 92% and 53%, respectively. Furthermore, lesions resected by ESD versus EMR demonstrated a recurrence rate of 0.3% versus 12%, respectively, with statistical significance.[9]

In a retrospective study of 274 difficult to treat colonic polyps, EMR was technically successful in achieving curative endoscopic resection in 91% of patients with a recurrence rate of 27%.[10] A meta-analysis including 8 studies and 2299 colonic lesions removed by EMR or ESD, the pooled odds ratio (OR) of curative resection, and recurrence rate for ESD versus EMR was 4.26 and 0.08, respectively.[5]

Although performing ESD procedures requires advanced training and yield potentially higher complication rates, improved outcomes such as reduced morbidity, lower recurrence rates of lesions, and lower costs continue to challenge the ongoing debate of performing these procedures.[11]

ADVERSE EVENTS OF ENDOSCOPIC RESECTION IN THE GENERAL POPULATION

Adverse events such as bleeding and perforation are notable risks when performing endoscopic resection procedures. Immediate or delayed bleeding has differing outcomes but is the most common complication that occurs postendoscopic resection. Delayed bleeding is defined as a decrease of over 2 g/dL of hemoglobin after remaining stable for the initial 24 hours postprocedure.

In the upper gastrointestinal tract, reported immediate bleeding postgastric polypectomies with either EMR or ESD range between 3.4% and 7.2%.[12,13] Similarly, delayed bleeding postpolypectomy of duodenal adenomas has been reported anywhere between 3.1% and 22%. In a previous meta-analysis by Cao and colleagues,[14] bleeding seems to have occurred more prominently in multifocal EMR as well as in EMR performed on gastric lesions. More recently, Burgess and colleagues[15] performed a large prospective study of 1172 patients who underwent upper gastrointestinal tract EMR with an overall incidence of perforation, bleeding, and strictures estimated between 0.5% and 5%.

A meta-analysis of 50 studies regarding endoscopic resection in the colon spanning from 1966 to 2014 reported rates of bleeding occurring in 423 out of 6474 patients (6.5%) who underwent colonic EMR.[16] However, an Australian prospective multicenter study of 479 patients that underwent EMR for colonic polyps greater than 20 mm reported bleeding in only 2.9%.[17]

Perforation rate vary according to the site of resection. Perforation rate following gastric ESD seems to be more frequent with ESD than EMR for gastric lesions. Significant risk factors for perforation included lesion size greater than 20 mm and procedure time greater than 2 hours.[18,19] A multicenter retrospective study of ESD procedures for gastric cancer yielded a statistically higher perforation rate after ESD than EMR: 4.5% versus 0.9%, respectively (OR 4.09, 95% confidence interval (CI): 2.47–6.80).[20] ESD procedures within the duodenum seem to have the highest risk of intraprocedural perforations, with a reported frequency of 33%[21] in the published data. In colorectal lesions undergoing ESD, perforation was reported in 10% of cases, and risk factors for perforations were related to lesion size and provider experience. However, only 0.5% of perforations required surgical intervention for the repair of the defects, highlighting significant advances in endoscopic closure and tissue apposition.[22] The heterogeneity between results from different studies may reflect differences in population age, location of lesions, comorbid conditions, and even operator experience. However, the overall estimated adverse events remain stable. Although the rate of adverse events in performing EMR and ESD procedures is higher in comparison to forceps polypectomies and cold snare polypectomies, one must consider that these procedures are performed for small lesions. Stricture formation is noted after the endoscopic resection of the large surface area, particularly after esophageal ESD when the resection area is greater than 75% of the esophageal circumference.[23]

OUTCOMES OF POLYPECTOMY, ENDOSCOPIC MUCOSAL RESECTION, AND ENDOSCOPIC SUBMUCOSAL DISSECTION IN PATIENTS WITH CIRRHOSIS
Adverse events in the lower gastrointestinal tract

In a recent retrospective cohort study of 1267 patients with chronic liver disease, immediate postpolypectomy bleeding (PPB) was significantly higher in the Child–Pugh (CP) B or C cirrhosis group (17.5%) compared with CP-A (6.3%) and chronic hepatitis (4.6%) groups (P<.001). Delayed PPB had similar outcomes too, with a delayed bleeding rate of 4.4% in the CP-B or C cirrhosis group compared with 0.7% in CP-A and 0.2% in chronic hepatitis groups (P<.001). Risk factors for bleeding in this study included a platelet count of less than 50,000/μL, the presence of 3 or more polyps, the use of EMR technique compared with standard polypectomy and endoscopic resection performed by trainees.[24] The finding of this study seems to be consistent with another study of 152 patients with chronic liver disease who underwent colonoscopy with polypectomy. In this study, delayed PPB was higher in cirrhotic patients versus patients with chronic hepatitis (13.8% vs 4.2%).[25] One must take into consideration that the mean prothrombin time was higher and the mean platelet count was lower in the CP-B, and CP-C group than chronic hepatitis and CP-A group. Data from another large retrospective cohort of cirrhotic patients by Kindumadam and colleagues[26] showed that the risk of PPB was 2% after 358 colonoscopies with polypectomy.

ADVERSE EVENTS IN THE UPPER GASTROINTESTINAL TRACT

In the upper gastrointestinal tract, there are scarce data regarding the safety and feasibility of performing polypectomies, EMR or ESD procedures. One large retrospective cohort study looked at 928 patients diagnosed with early gastric cancer or dysplasia in the setting of chronic renal failure (CRF) and cirrhosis who underwent endoscopic resections. Adverse events of immediate bleeding were found to be 47.5% in the CRF + cirrhosis group in comparison to 33.9% in the control group. This difference, however, did not achieve statistical significance. It appeared that the cohort with cirrhosis did not have a significantly higher bleeding risk in comparison to the control group. In a subgroup analysis regarding procedure methods, neither EMR nor ESD demonstrated a significantly higher complication rate when comparing ESD in the CRF + cirrhosis group versus EMR in the CRF + cirrhosis group, or ESD in the CRF + cirrhosis versus ESD and EMR in the control groups. This included a very small group of 40 patients from the entire cohort under investigation. It is noteworthy that most of those in the cirrhosis group were CP-A (72.2%). Although this was a small sample size, performing EMR and ESD for the management of early gastric neoplasia in patients with cirrhosis than healthy controls did not yield statistically significant adverse events.[27] Several studies have demonstrated the overall bleeding rates in cirrhotic patients undergoing ESD procedures between 4.3% and 16.7%.[27–30]

In patients with cirrhosis and early esophageal malignancies, a recent retrospective study of 40 patients with 50 superficial esophageal neoplasms undergoing ESD compared outcomes between those with underlying cirrhosis (8 patients) and a control group (32 patients). There were no reports of PPB or perforation in this study; however,

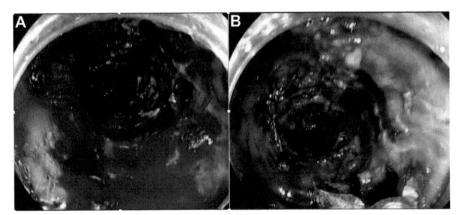

Fig. 1. Circumferential esophageal ESD in a cirrhotic patient with multifocal esophageal squamous cell carcinoma: (A) Post–ESD resection bleeding. (B) Bleeding control with coagulation grasper.

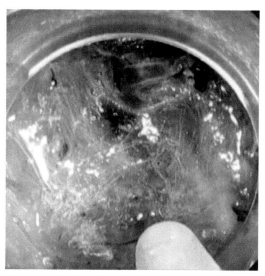

Fig. 2. Penetrating blood vessels identified in the submucosa during rectal ESD.

intraprocedural bleeding of statistical significance was noted in 2 cirrhotic patients with esophageal varices (18.2%) versus 0% in noncirrhotics.[31] In these circumstances, band ligation was performed for varices with sizes amenable to eradication or ESD was performed with the varices visible. Therefore, perhaps, if complete eradication of these varices were performed, it is possible that the small number of patients who developed intraprocedural bleeding may have decreased. **Fig. 1** shows circumferential esophageal ESD for squamous cell carcinoma with oozing submucosal blood vessels in a cirrhotic patient.

ENDOSCOPIC RESECTION IN CIRRHOTIC PATIENTS FROM THE AUTHORS' PERSPECTIVE

In our personal experience, performing ESD in cirrhotic patients is associated with frequent intraprocedural bleeding. However, ESD allows bleeding control in a careful manner using a coagulation grasper. To decrease the risk of PPB, the authors use a coagulation grasper with soft coagulation current (effect 5, 50 W) to treat any visible vessels in the postresection bed (**Fig. 2** shows penetrating blood vessels identified in the submucosa during rectal ESD). The authors strive to close postresection defects for all gastric and colonic lesions either with clips or endoscopic suturing. Prophylactic clipping post–EMR was shown to decrease PPB in a large multicenter trial.[32] ESD for esophageal and rectal lesions in the presence of varices is possible but requires significant experience to separate the lesion from underlying varices in the submucosa with meticulous dissection. Endoscopists should be ready to perform endoscopic band ligation in case of uncontrolled bleeding.

DISCLOSURE

A. Nakshabandi declares no conflict of interest with any commercial, financial, or funding sources.

M. O. Othman is a consultant for Olympus, Boston Scientific Corporation, Conmed, Apollo, Lumendi, and AbbVie. M. O. Othman had received research grants from Abb-Vie, Lumendi, and Lucid Diagnostics.

REFERENCES

1. Rosenberg N. Submucosal saline wheal as safety factor in fulguration or rectal and sigmoidal polypi. AMA Arch Surg 1955;70(1):120–2.
2. Fahrtash-Bahin F, Holt BA, Jayasekeran V, et al. Snare tip soft coagulation achieves effective and safe endoscopic hemostasis during wide-field endoscopic resection of large colonic lesions (with videos). Gastrointest Endosc 2013;78(1):158–63.e1.
3. Binmoeller KF, Weilert F, Shah J, et al. "Underwater" EMR without submucosal injection for large sessile colorectal polyps (with video). Gastrointest Endosc 2012; 75(5):1086–91.
4. Hirao M, Masuda K, Asanuma T, et al. Endoscopic resection of early gastric cancer and other tumors with local injection of hypertonic saline-epinephrine. Gastrointest Endosc 1988;34(3):264–9.
5. Fujiya M, Tanaka K, Dokoshi T, et al. Efficacy and adverse events of EMR and endoscopic submucosal dissection for the treatment of colon neoplasms: a meta-analysis of studies comparing EMR and endoscopic submucosal dissection. Gastrointest Endosc 2015;81(3):583–95.
6. Ning B, Abdelfatah MM, Othman MO. Endoscopic submucosal dissection and endoscopic mucosal resection for early stage esophageal cancer. Ann Cardiothorac Surg 2017;6(2):88–98.
7. Keihanian T, Othman MO. Colorectal endoscopic submucosal dissection: an Update on best practice. Clin Exp Gastroenterol 2021;14:317–30.
8. Ahlenstiel G, Hourigan LF, Brown G, et al. Actual endoscopic versus predicted surgical mortality for treatment of advanced mucosal neoplasia of the colon. Gastrointest Endosc 2014;80(4):668–76.
9. Komeda Y, Bruno M, Koch A. EMR is not inferior to ESD for early Barrett's and EGJ neoplasia: an extensive review on outcome, recurrence and complication rates. Endosc Int Open 2014;2(2):E58–64.
10. Buchner AM, Guarner-Argente C, Ginsberg GG. Outcomes of EMR of defiant colorectal lesions directed to an endoscopy referral center. Gastrointest Endosc 2012;76(2):255–63.
11. Yang D, Othman M, Draganov PV. Endoscopic mucosal resection vs endoscopic submucosal dissection for barrett's esophagus and colorectal neoplasia. Clin Gastroenterol Hepatol 2019;17(6):1019–28.
12. Inoue H, Minami H, Kaga M, et al. Endoscopic mucosal resection and endoscopic submucosal dissection for esophageal dysplasia and carcinoma. Gastrointest Endosc Clin N Am 2010;20(1):25–34, v–vi.
13. Seewald S, Ang TL, Gotoda T, et al. Total endoscopic resection of Barrett esophagus. Endoscopy 2008;40(12):1016–20.
14. Cao Y, Liao C, Tan A, et al. Meta-analysis of endoscopic submucosal dissection versus endoscopic mucosal resection for tumors of the gastrointestinal tract. Endoscopy 2009;41(9):751–7.
15. Burgess NG, Metz AJ, Williams SJ, et al. Risk factors for intraprocedural and clinically significant delayed bleeding after wide-field endoscopic mucosal resection of large colonic lesions. Clin Gastroenterol Hepatol 2014;12(4):651–61, e651–3.

16. Hassan C, Repici A, Sharma P, et al. Efficacy and safety of endoscopic resection of large colorectal polyps: a systematic review and meta-analysis. Gut 2016; 65(5):806–20.
17. Moss A, Bourke MJ, Williams SJ, et al. Endoscopic mucosal resection outcomes and prediction of submucosal cancer from advanced colonic mucosal neoplasia. Gastroenterology 2011;140(7):1909–18.
18. Nonaka S, Oda I, Makazu M, et al. Endoscopic submucosal dissection for early gastric cancer in the remnant stomach after gastrectomy. Gastrointest Endosc 2013;78(1):63–72.
19. Watari J, Tomita T, Toyoshima F, et al. Clinical outcomes and risk factors for perforation in gastric endoscopic submucosal dissection: a prospective pilot study. World J Gastrointest Endosc 2013;5(6):281–7.
20. Oda I, Saito D, Tada M, et al. A multicenter retrospective study of endoscopic resection for early gastric cancer. Gastric Cancer 2006;9(4):262–70.
21. Perez-Cuadrado-Robles E, Queneherve L, Margos W, et al. ESD versus EMR in non-ampullary superficial duodenal tumors: a systematic review and meta-analysis. Endosc Int Open 2018;6(8):E998–1007.
22. Lee EJ, Lee JB, Lee SH, et al. Endoscopic submucosal dissection for colorectal tumors–1,000 colorectal ESD cases: one specialized institute's experiences. Surg Endosc 2013;27(1):31–9.
23. Othman MO, Bahdi F, Ahmed Y, et al. Short-term clinical outcomes of non-curative endoscopic submucosal dissection for early esophageal adenocarcinoma. Eur J Gastroenterol Hepatol 2021. [Epub ahead of print].
24. Soh H, Chun J, Hong SW, et al. Child-pugh B or C cirrhosis Increases the risk for bleeding following colonoscopic polypectomy. Gut Liver 2020;14(6):755–64.
25. Lee HS, Park JJ, Kim SU, et al. Incidence and risk factors of delayed postpolypectomy bleeding in patients with chronic liver disease. Scand J Gastroenterol 2016;51(5):618–24.
26. Kundumadam S, Phatharacharukul P, Reinhart K, et al. Bleeding after elective interventional endoscopic procedures in a large cohort of patients with cirrhosis. Clin Transl Gastroenterol 2020;11(12):e00288.
27. Kwon YL, Kim ES, Lee KI, et al. Endoscopic treatments of gastric mucosal lesions are not riskier in patients with chronic renal failure or liver cirrhosis. Surg Endosc 2011;25(6):1994–9.
28. Ogura K, Okamoto M, Sugimoto T, et al. Efficacy and safety of endoscopic submucosal dissection for gastric cancer in patients with liver cirrhosis. Endoscopy 2008;40(5):443–5.
29. Kato M, Nishida T, Hamasaki T, et al. Outcomes of ESD for patients with early gastric cancer and comorbid liver cirrhosis: a propensity score analysis. Surg Endosc 2015;29(6):1560–6.
30. Choi JH, Kim ER, Min BH, et al. The feasibility and safety of the endoscopic submucosal dissection of superficial gastric neoplastic lesions in patients with compensated liver cirrhosis: a retrospective study. Gut Liver 2012;6(1):58–63.
31. Tsou Y-K, Liu C-Y, Fu K-I, et al. Endoscopic Submucosal Dissection of Superficial Esophageal Neoplasms Is Feasible and Not Riskier for Patients with Liver Cirrhosis. Dig Dis Sci 2016;61(12):3565–71.
32. Pohl H, Grimm IS, Moyer MT, et al. Clip closure prevents bleeding after endoscopic resection of large colon polyps in a Randomized trial. Gastroenterology 2019;157(4):977–84.e3.

Endoscopic Treatment of Esophageal Varices

Marc J. Zuckerman, MD*, Sherif Elhanafi, MD, Antonio Mendoza Ladd, MD

KEYWORDS

- Cirrhosis • Esophageal varices • Esophageal variceal bleeding
- Esophageal variceal banding • Esophageal variceal ligation
- Esophageal variceal sclerotherapy • Sengstaken-Blakemore tube

KEY POINTS

- Acute variceal bleeding is a serious complication of portal hypertension, usually due to cirrhosis, with high morbidity and mortality.
- Endoscopy plays a major role in the diagnosis and risk stratification of esophageal varices, but noninvasive tests including liver elastography also may be useful for screening.
- For the prevention of first variceal hemorrhage in patients with medium or large varices found on endoscopy, either nonselective β-blockers or endoscopic variceal ligation is recommended.
- For acute variceal bleed, the recommended type of endoscopic therapy is esophageal variceal ligation (banding). This should be repeated at intervals until eradication of esophageal varices to prevent rebleeding.
- For acute variceal bleeding refractory to standard pharmacologic and endoscopic therapy, bridge therapy with either a Sengstaken-Blakemore tube or a self-expanding covered metallic esophageal stent can be used.

INTRODUCTION

Esophageal varices (EVs) are a persistent global public health concern. Although the incidence of EVs varies widely, they remain one of the most common causes of acute upper gastrointestinal (GI) bleeding worldwide. Acute variceal bleeding (AVB) is a serious and often fatal complication of portal hypertension (PH). Its high morbidity and mortality, along with the costs associated with its treatment, pose serious problems from a public health perspective. This article presents an overview of the epidemiology, pathophysiology, prevention, and treatment of EV bleeding.

Division of Gastroenterology and Hepatology, Texas Tech University Health Sciences Center, 4800 Alberta Avenue, El Paso, TX 79905, USA
* Corresponding author.
E-mail address: Marc.Zuckerman@ttuhsc.edu

Clin Liver Dis 26 (2022) 21–37
https://doi.org/10.1016/j.cld.2021.08.003
1089-3261/22/© 2021 Elsevier Inc. All rights reserved.

liver.theclinics.com

EPIDEMIOLOGY

The global incidence of EVs is difficult to determine due to a variability among regions and the problem of underreporting. Recent statistics show that EVs are the seventh most common cause of GI bleeding in the United States.[1] In Africa, however, EVs are the leading cause due to high prevalence of schistosomiasis.[2] In the west, the most common cause of EVs is cirrhosis, and up to 85% of cirrhotic patients develop EVs at some point in their lives.[3–5] The incidence of EVs in cirrhosis depends on the severity of the disease. Compensated cirrhotics develop EVs at an annual rate of 8%,[6] but in decompensated cases the rate is higher. The distal third of the esophagus is the most common location of EVs, but proximal varices can be seen in conditions that affect extraportal venous circuits.[7,8]

The most feared complication of PH is AVB. It is estimated that one-third of patients with EVs develop AVB. The overall mortality associated with a first episode, however, ranges from 10% in compensated cirrhotics to 70% in those with decompensated disease.[5] The 6-week mortality of patients with an AVB is approximately 25%.[6,9] Once patients experience a first episode, their risk of rebleeding within 1 year is 80% and their 1-year mortality is 64%.[5] The overall severity and mortality of an AVB are associated directly with the severity of cirrhosis and the existence of comorbidities.

Management of AVB incurs considerable expense worldwide. In the United States alone, recent data show that the cost of hospitalization for AVB ranges approximately from $6000 to $23,000.[10] Considering that the most recent prevalence of cirrhosis in the United States was estimated to be 0.27%,[11] the total number of cirrhotic individuals currently in the country is approximately 894,000. Because approximately one-third of all cirrhotics develop AVB, the potential estimated cost of AVB in the country is $1.8 billion to $6.8 billion. These are alarming figures that demand better tactics for identification of cirrhotic patients at risk for AVB as well as prophylaxis.

PATHOPHYSIOLOGY

EVs develop in the presence of PH, which is defined by a portal pressure (PP) of greater than 5 mm Hg. Classically, the PP has been measured indirectly through the determination of the hepatic venous pressure gradient (HVPG). This is done by measuring the pressure of the hepatic vein (HV) in 2 separate scenarios. A balloon catheter is introduced through the jugular or femoral vein and advanced to the HV. With the balloon deflated, the pressure of the HV is measured while the catheter floats freely inside the vein. This establishes the HV pressure (FHVP). Once this is done, the balloon is inflated until the HV is completely occluded. This creates a column of fluid behind the balloon that determines the wedged HVP (WHVP). The HVPG is the difference between the WHVP and the FHVP and it represents the gradient between portal vein and the intra-abdominal vena cava pressure. The advantage of using the HVPG is that it is not affected by variations in intra-abdominal pressure.[12] Recently, a device to measure the PP directly was introduced to the market. This device is works via a 25-gauge needle that is inserted directly into the portal vein using endoscopic ultrasound guidance.[13,14]

The degree of PH is a major determinant of the EV bleeding risk. As a rule, it is widely accepted that EVs do not develop until the PP is greater than or equal to 10 mm Hg and that bleeding does not occur until it is greater than or equal to 12 mm Hg. The etiology of PH commonly is divided in 3 major groups: prehepatic, hepatic, and posthepatic. In cirrhosis, PP increases mostly due to an increase in the intrahepatic resistance to blood flow and to a nitrous oxide–induced splanchnic vasodilation. The vasodilation is not exclusive to the splanchnic circulation. Systemic vasodilation also occurs and leads to neurohumoral mechanisms that promote an intravascular volume increase. This creates a hyperdynamic circulatory state that increases flow through the portal system, thus worsening PH.[6] As a consequence, portosystemic collaterals develop in different venous circuits, such as the hemorrhoidal bed, the umbilical vein, and the coronary and short gastric veins (which lead to the formation of esophageal and gastric varices).

DIAGNOSIS AND RISK STRATIFICATION

The gold standard for the diagnosis of EVs is esophagogastroduodenoscopy (EGD). The advantages of EGD over other diagnostic methods include its ability to risk stratify through determining size and high-risk stigmata but most importantly its added therapeutic capacities. Whenever possible, EGD should be the preferred diagnostic and therapeutic tool of EV. In regions of the world where cost and availability limit the access to endoscopy, other methods can be used, but practitioners should understand that their performance is inferior and therefore should be cautious when interpreting their results. Physical examination may reveal evidence of PH (caput medusa, enlarged hemorrhoids, platypnea, orthodeoxia, or hepatosplenomegaly). The presence or absence of these signs and symptoms, however, do not necessarily correlate with the presence of EV. Doppler ultrasound can demonstrate collateral circulation or reversal of portal flow. Computed tomography and magnetic resonance imaging can demonstrate splenorenal shunts, dilated left and short gastric veins, and recanalization of the umbilical vein.

A noninvasive modality that has demonstrated promising results in risk stratification is liver elastography. Elastography provides a noninvasive assessment of the degree of liver stiffness. Studies have reported that in patients with compensated cirrhosis, liver stiffness paired with platelet count accurately identifies patients with a low (<5%) risk of EV.[15,16] These data have been obtained in patients with nonalcoholic steatohepatitis–induced cirrhosis as well as in cases secondary to viral hepatitis.[17,18] Baveno VI guidelines recommend it is not necessary to do upper endoscopy for patients with liver stiffness measurements below 20 kPa and platelet counts above 150,000 platelets μ/L of blood.[19] This was validated in a large cohort of patients with hepatitis B–associated and hepatitis C–associated cirrhosis in France.[18] Based on a large number of studies using elastography-based methods, this algorithm may be used to rule out varices needing treatment[20] Nonalcoholic fatty liver disease may be more variable than alcohol-induced or viral chronic liver disease,[21] and a more complex sequential algorithm incorporating etiology, sex, and international normalized ratio may be more useful. Although approximately 20% of endoscopies to rule out high-risk varices potentially could be avoided using noninvasive tests, in general, upper endoscopy is recommended to screen for varices.[22]

Artificial intelligence is rapidly positioning itself as a tool to minimize human errors in medicine. In a recent study, Chen and colleagues[23] explored the accuracy of endoscopy assistance with a convolutional neural network in detecting and risk stratifying EV. This included accurately differentiating large or small varices and red color signs. The investigators reported that this neural network outperformed human operators in both detection and risk stratification of EV. Artificial intelligence may have the potential to improve the accuracy of predicting risk factors for AVB.

Capsule endoscopy, using a specially developed esophageal capsule system, has been proposed as a modality for the diagnosis and grading of EVs in patients with PH. A meta-analysis of 17 studies found that capsule endoscopy was feasible and safe with a pooled diagnostic sensitivity of 83% and specificity of 85%.[24] The diagnostic accuracy for the grading of medium to large varices was 92%. The authors conclude that capsule endoscopy may have a role in patients with cirrhosis and suspicion of PH who otherwise refuse or have a contraindication to EGD.

The current recommendations by the American Association for the Study of Liver Diseases (AASLD) for the screening and monitoring of EVs in patients with compensated cirrhosis are listed in **Table 1**.[6] EGD is recommended annually for patients with decompensated cirrhosis.

PREVENTION OF FIRST ESOPHAGEAL VARICEAL HEMORRHAGE

There are 3 scenarios for the endoscopic management of EVs: role in the prevention of first variceal bleed, treatment of acute variceal hemorrhage, and secondary prophylaxis after a variceal bleed. Recommendations for prevention of first variceal hemorrhage are based on the AASLD guidelines[6] and the Baveno VI consensus workshop,[19] as well as guidelines of the American Society for Gastrointestinal Endoscopy (ASGE),[25] British Society of Gastroenterology (BSG),[26] and European Society of Gastrointestinal Endoscopy (ESGE).[27]

The AASLD recommends primary prophylaxis of variceal hemorrhage in patients at a high risk of bleeding: patients with medium/large varices, patients with small varices and red color signs, and decompensated patients with small varices[6] (**Figs. 1** and **2**).

The following is a summary of the guidelines.[27] In compensated patients with no varices at screening endoscopy and with ongoing liver injury (eg, alcohol use or active hepatitis C virus infection), surveillance endoscopy should be repeated at 2-year intervals. In compensated patients with small varices and with ongoing liver injury, surveillance endoscopy should be repeated at 1-year intervals. In compensated patients with no varices at screening endoscopy in whom the etiologic factor has been removed and who have no cofactors, surveillance endoscopy should be repeated at 3-year intervals. In patients with small varices with red wale marks or Child-Pugh class C, there is an increased risk of bleeding and they should be treated with a nonselective β-blocker (NSBB). Patients with small varices without signs of increased risk may be treated with NSBB to prevent bleeding.

In patients with medium or large varices, either NSBB or endoscopic variceal ligation (EVL) is recommended[27] (see **Table 1**). The choice of therapy should take note of patient characteristics, contraindications, and adverse events. The ASGE recommends EVL for patients who cannot tolerate β-blockers or who have contraindications to these agents as well as patients who have large varices with high-risk stigmata or Child-Pugh class B or class C cirrhosis. Studies have looked at comparison between endoscopic variceal sclerotherapy (EVS) and no treatment, between EVL and no treatment, between EVL and β-blockers, and between EVL and EVS.[28] Because EVS is associated with a higher frequency of complications, it is not recommended for the prevention of first variceal bleeding. Transjugular intrahepatic portosystemic shunts (TIPS) placement also is not recommended for the prevention of first variceal hemorrhage.[6]

Table 1		
Screening and surveillance intervals for endoscopy in patients with cirrhosis		
Esophageal Varices	Liver Injury Status	Endoscopy Interval
Absent	Quiescent	3 y
	Ongoing	2 y
Small	Quiescent	2 y
	Ongoing	1 y

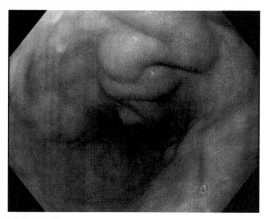

Fig. 1. EVs with no high-risk features.

For patients treated with EVL, repeat endoscopy is recommended every 2 weeks to 8 weeks until eradication of EV, with the first EGD performed 3 months to 6 months after eradication and then every 6 months to 12 months.[6,25] Combination therapy with EVL and β-blockers is not recommended for primary prophylaxis because it has not been shown to decrease bleeding risk or mortality and is associated with increased side-effects. PPI usually are used as adjunctive therapy to reduce the risk of ligation-induced ulcers.[25]

ENDOSCOPIC TREATMENTS FOR ACUTE ESOPHAGEAL VARICEAL HEMORRHAGE AND PREVENTION OF REBLEEDING

Recommendations for the treatment and prevention of recurrence of AVB are based primarily on consensus conferences and major gastroenterology and hepatology societies, including the Baveno VI consensus workshop[19] and the AASLD,[6] as well as the ASGE,[25] BSG,[26] and ESGE.[27] The ESGE guidelines[27] use a cascade approach to resource-sensitive statements from the Baveno VI guidelines.

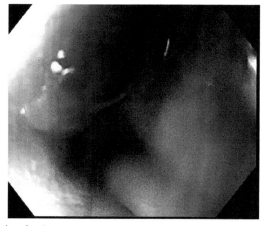

Fig. 2. EVs with red wale sign.

Patients presenting with AVB are considered decompensated, with a 5-year mortality of at least 20% and much greater if there are multiple complications of cirrhosis.[6] Child-Pugh class helps with risk stratification. Goals of therapy include control of bleeding, preventing early recurrence of bleeding, and reducing the 6-week mortality outcome.

General Management of Acute Variceal Bleeding

Management of AVB includes blood volume resuscitation, antibiotic prophylaxis, prevention of hepatic encephalopathy, pharmacologic treatment with vasoactive drugs, and endoscopy.[6,27] Standard endoscopic therapy is with EVL or alternatively EVS (**Table 2**). Injection of tissue adhesive agents and spraying hemostatic powder (HPs) have been tried but commonly are reserved for AVB that cannot be controlled by standard interventions.[28] Cases of AVB refractory to standard endoscopic therapy may be treated with balloon tamponade (BT), placement of esophageal stents, or TIPS.

The AASLD recommends[6] volume resuscitation to maintain hemodynamic stability and restrictive blood transfusion. In general, the target for transfusion of packed red blood cells is 7 g/dL to 8 g/dL but is individualized based on age and cardiac and hemodynamic status. Correction of coagulopathy has been controversial and the use of fresh frozen plasma to correct the INR is not recommended, Routine use of platelet transfusion also is not specified.[27] Antibiotic prophylaxis after obtaining blood cultures is recommended due to the high risk of infections in cirrhotics presenting with GI bleeding. Antibiotic prophylaxis with ceftriaxone, 1 g once daily, commonly is recommended, for a maximum of 7 days. Vasoactive drugs have been shown to improve control of acute hemorrhage. Octreotide, terlipressin, and somatostatin are the recommended vasoactive drugs for the management of AVB with no significant differences in major outcomes, but somatostatin and octreotide have better safety profiles.[19] Octreotide is used in the United States and generally is given as an initial intravenous bolus of 50 μg followed by a continuous infusion of 50 μg/h for 3 days to 5 days. The mechanism of vasoactive drugs for variceal bleeding control, unlike direct hemostasis with endoscopy, is reduction in HVPG. Vasoactive drugs have been shown to decrease 7-day mortality and transfusion requirements.[29] The optimal adjuvant vasoactive drugs regimen of 3-day to 5-day duration may not be associated with less early rebleeding or mortality than a shorter course.[30]

Timing of Endoscopy and Diagnosis of Acute Variceal Bleeding

Guidelines recommend that patients with suspected AVB undergo EGD within 12 hours of presentation.[6,19,25,27] Endoscopy usually is performed with protection

Table 2
Modalities for endoscopic treatment of esophageal varices

Modality	Active Bleed	Prevent Recurrence	Primary Prevention
Banding	Preferred	Preferred	Option
Sclerotherapy	Option	Option	No
SB tube	Salvage—may be placed endoscopically	No	No
Esophageal stent	Salvage—may be placed endoscopically	No	No
Hemostatic powder	Controversial	No	No

Note: nonendoscopic modalities include TIPS, surgical shunt.
Pharmacotherapy with nonselective β-blockers generally is given for primary prophylaxis.

of the airway in patients with active bleeding or altered consciousness due to the risk of aspiration. Diagnosis of AVB by endoscopy may be either certain or presumptive.[6] It is certain when active bleeding or a sign of recent bleeding is observed. It is presumptive when blood is present in the stomach and EVs are the only lesions found. Endoscopic treatment is indicated if an EV source either is confirmed or presumptive.

Endoscopic Variceal Ligation

Technique of endoscopic variceal ligation

The current technique for EVL uses a multiband device.[29,31] A cap-assisted ligation device on the endoscope is used to deploy an elastic band around a varix after it is suctioned into the cap, by turning a firing device attached at the external biopsy valve port. This causes varix strangulation and achieves hemostasis followed by intravascular thrombus formation, necrosis, and eventual fibrosis and obliteration of varices. Bands initially are placed distally and preferentially targeting varices with stigmata of recent hemorrhage, platelet plug (**Fig. 3**), or active bleeding (**Fig. 4**). Helical placement of bands is done distal to proximal. In the presence of active bleeding, this may be difficult due to impaired visualization.

Indications for endoscopic variceal ligation

EVL, or banding, is the recommended type of endoscopic therapy for AVB.[6,19,25–27] It was introduced in approximately 1986.[32] EVL is effective in immediate control of active variceal bleeding in approximately 90% of cases.[31] Many randomized controlled trials[28,33,34] since have compared the efficacy of EVL to EVS for AVB and a meta-analysis showed that EVL compared with EVS had lower rebleeding and mortality rates.[34] A more recent meta-analysis[35] found that EVL was better than EVS in terms of lower rate of rebleeding, complications, and higher rate of variceal eradication but no significant difference in mortality.

After the treatment of AVB, EVL should be repeated at intervals until varices are eradicated. The AASLD recommends intervals of 1 week to 4 weeks until eradication, often 2 sessions to 4 sessions, with the first follow-up EGD performed 3 months to 6 months after eradication and then every 6 months to 12 months.[6,25] Other investigators recommend elective EVL at 4-week to 6-week intervals.[29] Endoscopic ultrasound probe findings after EV eradication may be useful to predict variceal recurrence. A

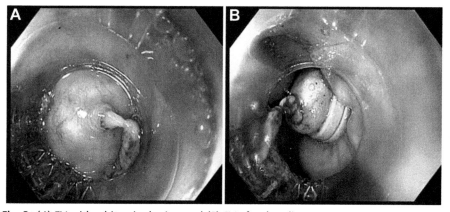

Fig. 3. (A) EV with white nipple sign and (B) EV after banding.

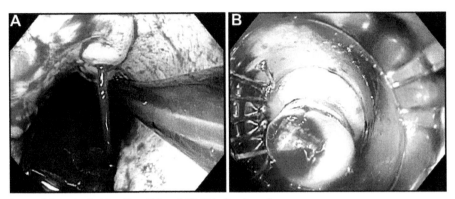

Fig. 4. (*A*) Actively bleeding EV and (*B*) EV after banding.

prospective cohort study using endoscopic ultrasound probe sonography showed potential for clinical application for the evaluation of EVs.[36]

Due to the high rebleeding risk after initial AVB (60%), combination therapy of NSBB (propranolol or nadolol) is recommended, because this has been demonstrated to be superior to EVL alone.[6,19] Recent data from meta-analyses show EVL is superior to EVS for secondary prophylaxis and that use of β-blockers combined with EVL reduces rebleeding rate.[37] EVL may be used alone if the patient cannot tolerate NSBB or if there is a contraindication to its use.[37]

If patients rebleed despite combination therapy with EVs and NSBB, TIPS is the recommended rescue treatment, taking into account the severity of rebleeding and other complications of PH, especially hepatic encephalopathy.[37,38] EVL and NSBB can be discontinued after successful TIPS placement.[29]

Complications of banding

Complications of EVL occur in 2% to 20% of patients and include transient dysphagia, retrosternal pain, postbanding bleeding, esophageal stricture, esophageal ulcerations, esophageal perforation and infection[31] (**Fig. 5**). Rebleeding may occur due to either recurrent variceal bleed or postbanding ulceration. Postbanding ulcer bleeding

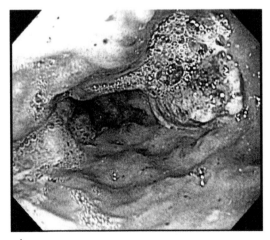

Fig. 5. Postbanding ulcer.

occurs in 3.6% to 15% of patients.[39] In an observational study, EVL-induced ulcer bleeding occurred in 7.7% of patients, with a mortality rate of 27.3%. Bleeding may be managed conservatively with PPI therapy and supportive care, but other options tried include repeat EVL, cyanoacrylate injection, argon plasma coagulation, and emergency TIPS as well as self-expanding metal stent (SEMS) placement and application HP. ASGE recommends to consider PPI as adjunctive therapy postbanding to potentially decrease the risk of bleeding.[25]

Although there have been reports of infection with both EVL and EVS, the incidence of transient bacteremia following EVL (3%–6%) may be lower than after EVS (0%–53%),[40–42] and the incidence of all types of infectious adverse events after EVL (1.8%) also may be lower than for EVS (18%).[41] Limitations of the studies of bacteremia after endoscopic variceal therapy are the difficulty of distinguishing significant from nonsignificant blood culture results and that most of the EVL studies used the older single banding technique rather than the current multiband ligating devices.

Esophageal Variceal Sclerotherapy

Technique of esophageal variceal sclerotherapy
The technique of EVL uses a catheter with a needle delivery device inserted through the endoscope port during endoscopy and does not require withdrawal of the endoscope to load the device. Agents used for sclerotherapy include sodium tetradecyl sulfate, ethanolamine oleate, sodium morrhuate, polidocanol, or absolute alcohol.[31] Intravariceal injection may be performed just distal to the site of bleeding or a paravariceal injection may be performed immediately adjacent to a varix. The sclerosant precipitates inflammation and thrombosis. This mechanism is more chemical as opposed to EVL, which is mechanical.[28] After injection near the bleeding site, injections are performed starting at all varices at the GE junction, with proximal injections at 2-cm intervals, extending up to 5 cm to 6 cm from the gastroesophageal junction.[43] Subsequent elective sclerotherapy sessions then are performed until eradication of varices, with more frequent treatment intervals associated with faster eradication. More frequent intervals are associated, however, with more local complications, such as ulceration.[25]

Indications for esophageal variceal sclerotherapy
EVS was the first endoscopic treatment shown to be superior to BT or vasoactive medication in the treatment of EV.[31,44] It commonly was used prior to the introduction of EVL. EVS controlled AVB in more than 90% of patients and was shown to reduce the frequency of recurrent variceal hemorrhage. Although endoscopic therapy initially was performed with EVS in the 1980s, it largely was replaced in the 1990s by EVL after studies showed there was fewer rebleeding episodes and adverse events.[28,45]

Although EVL is the first-choice treatment of AVB, there are certain situations where EVS may have a role. EVS is a potential option for patients in whom EVL is technically difficult.[19,25] At times, significant bleeding may impair visualization or scar tissue may prevent adequate suction of varices.[31] EVS may be useful in the setting of active bleeding in order to control bleeding prior to banding varices.[29] Rarely, there is a mechanical reason the endoscope with the banding device loaded on the tip is difficult to insert (eg, after cervical spine surgery), but the endoscope alone passes and allows a through-the-scope injection technique to be performed.

Combination therapy for EVL and EVS has not been shown to be better than EVL alone. A meta-analysis comparing EVL alone with EVL plus EVS as therapy for prevention of rebleeding found that the addition of therapy did not improve rebleeding rate, number of sessions, or mortality but had higher rates of esophageal stricture.[46] The consensus is that combined therapy does not have a role in the treatment of EV,[45] but some endoscopists use EVS after EVL because a type of salvage therapy if EVL alone does not sufficiently control bleeding (**Fig. 6**).

Complications of sclerotherapy

Complications of sclerotherapy occur in up to 40% of patients and include fever, dysphagia, retrosternal discomfort, injection-induced bleeding, esophageal ulceration with bleeding, esophageal stricture, esophageal perforation, pleural effusion, pneumothorax, mediastinitis, and infection (including spontaneous bacterial peritonitis).[25,43] Rebleeding may occur due to recurrent variceal bleed or to postinjection ulceration. Compared with EVL, EVS has been associated with a higher risk of complications, including pleuropulmonary complications, bleeding, and infection.[42] There have been reports of transient bacteremia after EVS but also after EVL. In a meta-analysis of studies of bacteremia after variceal therapy, it was found that the frequency of bacteremia after endoscopic variceal therapy was 13% overall, with the frequency of bacteremia after EVS (17%) showing a trend toward being higher than after EVL (6%). It also was found that the frequency of bacteremia after emergency EVS (22%) was significantly greater than after elective EVS (14%), but the frequency of bacteremia after emergency EVL (3.2%) was not significantly different from after elective EVL (7.6%).[47]

Endoscopic Tissue Adhesive

Endoscopic injection of tissue adhesive (ETA) is another method of treating varices, with few studies reporting its use in AVB.[48–50] It has been used more in the context of gastric varices and ectopic varices than with EVs. Endoscopic injection of tissue adhesive (cyanoacrylate tissue glue) causes endothelial injury and venous obturation leading to hemostasis.[51] A single-center retrospective study of patients with Child-Pugh class C cirrhosis and AVB treated with ETA (cyanoacrylate) found that bleeding was controlled successfully in approximately 75% of patients, with an overall mortality of 44%.[50] A single-center prospective study of patients with cirrhosis and AVB, not amenable to EVL due to profuse bleeding, randomly treated with either EVS or ETA found initial bleeding control was significantly higher with ETA with no significant difference in rebleeding rate. The investigators concluded that both EVS and ETA should be considered in patients with AVB when EVL is technically difficult. Standard

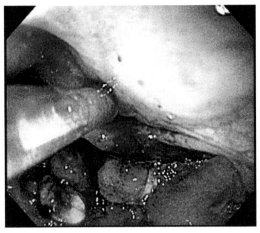

Fig. 6. Sclerotherapy for bleeding EVs after banding.

guidelines[6,19,26] recommend against the use of ETA as standard therapy for AVB. Complications include stricture formation and systemic embolism.

Hemostatic Powder

HPs can be administered endoscopically by spray through a specialized catheter-based delivery system. Hemospray (Cook Medical, Bloomington, Indiana) is an inert mineral based compound that absorbs water when in contact with blood and becomes adherent to the bleeding site. It can be administered by spraying from the upper part of the stomach up to the midthird of the esophagus for the purpose of treating EVs but has mainly been studied for use in ulcer bleeding and tumor bleeding. In a study of GI bleeding using either Hemospray or EndoClot (Micro-Tech Europe, Düsseldorf, Germany), 13 (7%) of patients treated had varices. There was an overall short-term success of 85% and long-term success of 56%[52] A trial of cirrhotic patients with AVB randomized to either early (<2 hours) application of HP followed by early elective endoscopy on the next day, compared with early elective endoscopy (12–24 hours), found a significant improvement in achieving hemostasis. The Baveno VI guidelines[19] consider alternative hemostasis techniques, such as HPs, as part of the research agenda to be studied for treating AVB. Another area of potential use for HPs is for treating postbanding ulcer bleeding.[39]

Refractory Bleeding

AVB may be unresponsive to standard medical therapy in 10% to 20% of cases. This may be due to either massive bleeding precluding endoscopic therapy or to failure to control bleeding or early rebleeding despite initial endoscopic and pharmacologic therapy. This is associated with a high mortality of approximately 30% to 50%.[6,53] Cases of AVB refractory to standard endoscopic therapy may be treated with BT, placement of esophageal stents, or TIPS. BT and esophageal stents are considered bridge therapy until rescue TIPS is performed.

Balloon tamponade

BT was introduced as a means to control AVB[54] and has been recommended for temporary control of bleeding for refractory AVB until more definitive therapy can be performed with either repeat endoscopy or TIPS.[6,25] BT with Sengstaken-Blakemore (SB) tube is used to mechanically tamponade varices in intubated patients[29] after endoscopy is performed. At times, an SB tube may be inserted when patients are too unstable to have endoscopy. SB tubes are generally left in place for only 24 hours.

BT is successful in approximately 80% to 90% of cases, but there is a high bleeding rate of approximately 50% once the balloon is deflated and a mortality of approximately 20%.[6] There have been some more recent reports of outcomes after BT. In a retrospective study of 34 patients with BT following AVB, 59% survived until discharge and of these, 95% had undergone TIPS.[55] In a retrospective cohort study of 66 patients with rescue therapy by BT, hemostasis was achieved in 75.8% with rebleeding in 22% and mortality of 24% in patients who achieved initial control.[56]

Various techniques have been described besides the original blind placement technique. It has been recommended that the SB tube be inflated only under direct vision to be sure it is in the stomach and that the esophageal balloon not be used.[4] An endoscopic grasp-and-place technique has been reported recently[57] (**Fig. 7**). To briefly describe the technique, after the initial endoscopy identifies the location of the variceal bleed not amenable to endoscopic therapy, the endoscope is withdrawn. A snare is introduced through the endoscope channel until it reaches the end of the endoscope and then the SB tube is snared at the tip of the endoscope and aligned along the side

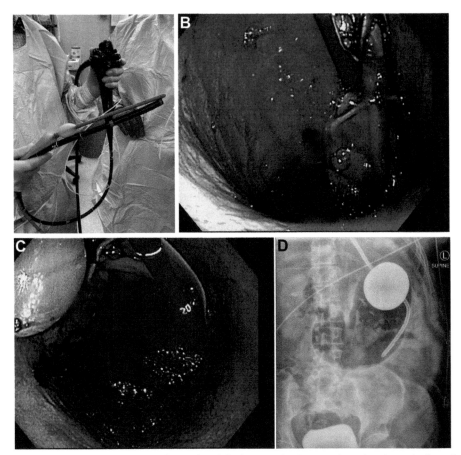

Fig. 7. Endoscopic placement of SB tube. (*A*) The SB tube is snared at the tip and aligned along the side of the endoscope; (*B*) introduction with retroflexed view of SB tube; (*C*) filling of balloon in retroflexed view; and (*D*) radiograph confirmation of SB tube placement.

of the endoscope. Then, both the endoscope and the SB tube are lubricated and inserted through the mouth as a single unit, holding both the endoscope and the tube together while advancing both simultaneously. The endoscope and the tube are advanced to the antrum and the SB tube then is detached from the snare and the snare removed. The endoscope then can be retroflexed to confirm correct positioning with direct visualization of the gastric balloon, which then is inflated with 50-mL diluted diatrizoate water soluble contrast agent while the endoscope is in the stomach. The endoscope can be withdrawn after the gastric balloon is inflated, carefully, in a spiral manner to avoid accidental removal of the SB tube. Once the endoscope is withdrawn, the gastric balloon can be inflated fully and traction applied. A radiograph can be taken prior to full inflation of the gastric balloon, and always should be taken postprocedure to confirm position.

Esophageal stents

SEMSs are an endoscopic alternative to BT for refractory or uncontrolled bleeding.[31] Stent placement then can be a bridge therapy to either EVL or TIPS. They can achieve hemostasis by direct compression of the varices. There have been case reports and more recently systematic reviews and meta-analyses using various stents. A specific stent system (SX-Ella Danis stent [Ella-CS, Hradec Kralove, Czech Republic]) was designed for AVB, which is a removable, covered, self-expanding nitinol metal stent with atraumatic edges that is placed with endoscopic guidance.[31] It can be left in place for up to 14 days.

A systematic review of and meta-analysis of 5 studies with the specialized SEMSs found stent deployed successfully in 96.7% of patients with refractory AVB, with hemostasis rate of 93.9% and rebleeding rate after stent of 13.2%.[58] Another systematic review and meta-analysis of 12 studies with the specialized SEMS and 2 other types of stent found technical success in 97% and achieved hemostasis in 96%.[59] A more recent retrospective multicenter study[60] of the specialized stent for refractory AVB found that SEMSs controlled bleeding in 79.4% of patients, 38.2% died with the stent in place, and bleeding related mortality was 47.1%.

One small randomized controlled trial with 28 patients compared the specialized SEMSs with BT in patients with cirrhosis and AVB refractory to pharmacologic and endoscopic treatment,[53] finding the stent more effective with control of bleeding in 85% versus 47%, combined success endpoint with stent placement 66% compared with BT 20%, and associated with lower transfusion requirements and adverse effects but no difference in mortality at 6 weeks. A systematic review and meta-analysis looking at both BT and esophageal stenting for AVB[61] found that BT had a pooled short-term failure to control bleeding rate of 35.5%, with adverse events in more than 20%, whereas stenting had less to control bleeding in the short term and medium term (12.7% and 21.7%), with stent migration in 23.8%. Mortality rates were similar in both groups. Additionally, stents are more comfortable than SB tubes, they may remain in place longer, and the patient may be able to eat while a stent is in place. Most studies conclude that esophageal stenting may be a better and safer bridge option than BT for refractory AVB.

A limitation of the esophageal stent studies is that the specialized stent is not available in the United States and results may not be generalizable to other types of esophageal stents.[62] The main complication seen is stent migration, but esophageal ulceration may occur as well.[60]

Transjugular intrahepatic portosystemic shunts

TIPS may have a role as early preemptive strategy to reduce rebleeding risk and as rescue modality. TIPS is recommended for patients with AVB refractory to endoscopic and pharmacologic therapy.[6,25,38] Early TIPS may be recommended for patients with AVB and high-risk features, patients who are Child-Pugh class B or Child-Pugh class C (score 10–13), or patients with Model for End-Stage Liver Disease greater than or equal to 19, who are hemodynamically stable.[38,48,63] TIPS also should be considered when patients rebleed despite combination of EVL and NSBB.[38] Patients who have a TIPS placed successfully during AVB do not require NSSBs or EVL.[6]

SUMMARY

Although EVL is the first-choice treatment of AVB, there are certain situations where EVS may have a role. Treatment with either an SB tube or a self-expanding covered metallic esophageal stent can be used for AVB refractory to standard pharmacologic and endoscopic therapy. SB tube placement can be done with endoscopic assistance. BT and esophageal stents are considered bridge therapy until rescue TIPS is performed.

CLINICS CARE POINTS

- Patients with cirrhosis should be screened for EVs. EVs screening and surveillance intervals for upper endoscopy in patients with cirrhosis have been recommended.
- EV ligation is an option for the prevention of first variceal hemorrhage in patients with medium or large varices found on endoscopy.
- The recommended type of endoscopic therapy for AVB is EV ligation (banding). This should be repeated at intervals until eradication of EVs to prevent rebleeding.
- Although banding is the first-choice treatment of AVB, there are certain situations where sclerotherapy may have a role.
- Bridge therapy with either an SB tube or a self-expanding covered metallic esophageal stent can be used for AVB refractory to standard pharmacologic and endoscopic therapy. SB tube placement can be done with endoscopic assistance.

DISCLOSURE

The authors have nothing to disclose.

REFERENCES

1. Wuerth BA, Rockey DC. Changing epidemiology of upper gastrointestinal hemorrhage in the last decade: a nationwide analysis. Dig Dis Sci 2018;63(5):1286–93.
2. Opio CK, Rejani L, Kazibwe F, et al. The diagnostic accuracy of routine clinical findings for detection of esophageal varices in rural sub-Saharan Africa where schistosomiasis is endemic. Afr Health Sci 2019;19(4):3225–34.
3. Nusrat S, Khan MS, Fazili J, et al. Cirrhosis and its complications: evidence based treatment. World J Gastroenterol 2014;20(18):5442–60.
4. Haq I, Tripathi D. Recent advances in the management of variceal bleeding. Gastroenterol Rep (Oxf) 2017;5(2):113–26.
5. LaBrecque D, Khan A, Sarin S, et al. Esophageal varices. World Gastroenterol Organ Glob Guidel 2014;2014:1–14.
6. Garcia-Tsao G, Abraldes JG, Berzigotti A, et al. Portal hypertensive bleeding in cirrhosis: risk stratification, diagnosis, and management: 2016 practice guidance by the American Association for the study of liver diseases. Hepatology 2017;65(1):310–35.
7. Rhoades DP, Forde KA, Tabibian JH. Proximal esophageal varices: a rare yet treatable cause of hemorrhage. Clin Gastroenterol Hepatol 2016;14(9):e105–6.
8. Areia M, Romãozinho JM, Ferreira M, et al. Downhill" varices. A rare cause of esophageal hemorrhage. Rev Esp Enferm Dig 2006;98(5):359–61.
9. Reverter E, Tandon P, Augustin S, et al. A MELD-based model to determine risk of mortality among patients with acute variceal bleeding. Gastroenterology 2014;146(2):412–9.e3.
10. Adam V, Barkun AN, Viviane A, et al. Estimates of costs of hospital stay for variceal and nonvariceal upper gastrointestinal bleeding in the United States. Value Health 2008;11(1):1–3.
11. Scaglione S, Kliethermes S, Cao G, et al. The epidemiology of cirrhosis in the United States: a Population-based study. J Clin Gastroenterol 2015;49(8):690–6.
12. Groszmann RJ, Wongcharatrawee S. The hepatic venous pressure gradient: anything worth doing should be done right. Hepatology 2004;39(2):280–3.

13. Trikudanathan G, Pannala R, Bhutani MS, et al. EUS-guided portal vein interventions. Gastrointest Endosc 2017;85(5):883–8.
14. Samarasena JB, Chang KJ. Endoscopic ultrasound-guided interventions for the measurement and treatment of portal hypertension. Gastrointest Endosc Clin N Am 2019;29(2):311–20.
15. Ding NS, Nguyen T, Iser DM, et al. Liver stiffness plus platelet count can be used to exclude high-risk oesophageal varices. Liver Int 2016;36(2):240–5.
16. Robic MA, Procopet B, Métivier S, et al. Liver stiffness accurately predicts portal hypertension related complications in patients with chronic liver disease: a prospective study. J Hepatol 2011;55(5):1017–24.
17. Kim BK, Han KH, Park JY, et al. A liver stiffness measurement-based, noninvasive prediction model for high-risk esophageal varices in B-viral liver cirrhosis. Am J Gastroenterol 2010;105(6):1382–90.
18. Thabut D, Bureau C, Layese R, et al. Validation of Baveno VI criteria for screening and surveillance of esophageal varices in patients with compensated cirrhosis and a sustained response to antiviral therapy. Gastroenterology 2019;156(4): 997–1009.e5.
19. de Franchis R. Expanding consensus in portal hypertension: report of the Baveno VI Consensus Workshop: stratifying risk and individualizing care for portal hypertension. J Hepatol 2015;63(3):743–52.
20. Paternostro R, Reiberger T, Bucsics T. Elastography-based screening for esophageal varices in patients with advanced chronic liver disease. World J Gastroenterol 2019;25(3):308–29.
21. Berger A, Ravaioli F, Farcau O, et al. Including ratio of platelets to liver stiffness improves accuracy of screening for esophageal varices that require treatment. Clin Gastroenterol Hepatol 2021;19(4):777–87.e17.
22. Turco L, Garcia-Tsao G. Portal hypertension: Pathogenesis and diagnosis. Clin Liver Dis 2019;23(4):573–87.
23. Chen M, Wang J, Xiao Y, et al. Automated and real-time validation of gastro-esophageal varices under esophagogastroduodenoscopy using a deep convolutional neural network: a multicenter retrospective study (with video). Gastrointest Endosc 2021;93(2):422–32.e3.
24. McCarty TR, Afinogenova Y, Njei B. Use of wireless capsule endoscopy for the diagnosis and grading of esophageal varices in patients with portal hypertension: a systematic review and meta-analysis. J Clin Gastroenterol 2017;51(2):174–82.
25. Hwang JH, Shergill AK, Acosta RD, et al. The role of endoscopy in the management of variceal hemorrhage. Gastrointest Endosc 2014;80(2):221–7.
26. Tripathi D, Stanley AJ, Hayes PC, et al. U.K. guidelines on the management of variceal haemorrhage in cirrhotic patients. Gut 2015;64(11):1680–704.
27. Karstensen JG, Ebigbo A, Bhat P, et al. Endoscopic treatment of variceal upper gastrointestinal bleeding: European society of gastrointestinal endoscopy (ESGE) cascade guideline. Endosc Int Open 2020;8(7):E990–7.
28. Lo GH. Endoscopic treatments for portal hypertension. Hepatol Int 2018; 12(Suppl 1):91–101.
29. Kovacs TOG, Jensen DM. Varices: esophageal, gastric, and rectal. Clin Liver Dis 2019;23(4):625–42.
30. Yan P, Tian X, Li J. Is additional 5-day vasoactive drug therapy necessary for acute variceal bleeding after successful endoscopic hemostasis?: a systematic review and meta-analysis. Medicine (Baltimore) 2018;97(41):e12826.
31. Nett A, Binmoeller KF. Endoscopic management of portal hypertension-related bleeding. Gastrointest Endosc Clin N Am 2019;29(2):321–37.

32. Van Stiegmann G, Cambre T, Sun JH. A new endoscopic elastic band ligating device. Gastrointest Endosc 1986;32(3):230–3.

33. Stiegmann GV, Goff JS, Michaletz-Onody PA, et al. Endoscopic sclerotherapy as compared with endoscopic ligation for bleeding esophageal varices. N Engl J Med 1992;326(23):1527–32.

34. Laine L, Cook D. Endoscopic ligation compared with sclerotherapy for treatment of esophageal variceal bleeding. A meta-analysis. Ann Intern Med 1995;123(4): 280–7.

35. Dai C, Liu WX, Jiang M, et al. Endoscopic variceal ligation compared with endoscopic injection sclerotherapy for treatment of esophageal variceal hemorrhage: a meta-analysis. World J Gastroenterol 2015;21(8):2534–41.

36. Zheng J, Zhang Y, Li P, et al. The endoscopic ultrasound probe findings in prediction of esophageal variceal recurrence after endoscopic variceal eradication therapies in cirrhotic patients: a cohort prospective study. BMC Gastroenterol 2019;19(1):32.

37. Aggeletopoulou I, Konstantakis C, Manolakopoulos S, et al. Role of band ligation for secondary prophylaxis of variceal bleeding. World J Gastroenterol 2018; 24(26):2902–14.

38. Tripathi D, Stanley AJ, Hayes PC, et al. Transjugular intrahepatic portosystemic stent-shunt in the management of portal hypertension. Gut 2020;69(7):1173–92.

39. Cho E, Jun CH, Cho SB, et al. Endoscopic variceal ligation-induced ulcer bleeding: what are the risk factors and treatment strategies? Medicine (Baltimore) 2017;96(24):e7157.

40. Ho H, Zuckerman MJ, Wassem C. A prospective controlled study of the risk of bacteremia in emergency sclerotherapy of esophageal varices. Gastroenterology 1991;101(6):1642–8.

41. Lo GH, Lai KH, Shen MT, et al. A comparison of the incidence of transient bacteremia and infectious sequelae after sclerotherapy and rubber band ligation of bleeding esophageal varices. Gastrointest Endosc 1994;40(6):675–9.

42. Zuckerman MJ, Jia Y, Hernandez JA, et al. A prospective randomized study on the risk of bacteremia in banding versus sclerotherapy of esophageal varices. Front Med (Lausanne) 2016;3:16.

43. Kapoor A, Dharel N, Sanyal AJ. Endoscopic diagnosis and therapy in gastroesophageal variceal bleeding. Gastrointest Endosc Clin N Am 2015;25(3): 491–507.

44. Westaby D, Macdougall BR, Melia W, et al. A prospective randomized study of two sclerotherapy techniques for esophageal varices. Hepatology 1983;3(5): 681–4.

45. Laine L. Is there a role for combined sclerotherapy and ligation in the endoscopic treatment of gastroesophageal varices? Gastrointest Endosc 2017;86(2):316–8.

46. Karsan HA, Morton SC, Shekelle PG, et al. Combination endoscopic band ligation and sclerotherapy compared with endoscopic band ligation alone for the secondary prophylaxis of esophageal variceal hemorrhage: a meta-analysis. Dig Dis Sci 2005;50(2):399–406.

47. Jia Y, Dwivedi A, Elhanafi S, et al. Low risk of bacteremia after endoscopic variceal therapy for esophageal varices: a systematic review and meta-analysis. Endosc Int Open 2015;3(5):E409–17.

48. Nevens F, Bittencourt PL, Coenraad MJ, et al. Recommendations on the diagnosis and initial management of acute variceal bleeding and Hepatorenal syndrome in patients with cirrhosis. Dig Dis Sci 2019;64(6):1419–31.

49. Cipolletta L, Zambelli A, Bianco MA, et al. Acrylate glue injection for acutely bleeding oesophageal varices: a prospective cohort study. Dig Liver Dis 2009; 41(10):729–34.
50. Ribeiro JP, Matuguma SE, Cheng S, et al. Results of treatment of esophageal variceal hemorrhage with endoscopic injection of n-butyl-2-cyanoacrylate in patients with Child-Pugh class C cirrhosis. Endosc Int Open 2015;3(6):E584–9.
51. Al-Khazraji A, Curry MP. The current knowledge about the therapeutic use of endoscopic sclerotherapy and endoscopic tissue adhesives in variceal bleeding. Expert Rev Gastroenterol Hepatol 2019;13(9):893–7.
52. Vitali F, Naegel A, Atreya R, et al. Comparison of Hemospray(®) and Endoclot(™) for the treatment of gastrointestinal bleeding. World J Gastroenterol 2019;25(13): 1592–602.
53. Escorsell À, Pavel O, Cárdenas A, et al. Esophageal balloon tamponade versus esophageal stent in controlling acute refractory variceal bleeding: a multicenter randomized, controlled trial. Hepatology 2016;63(6):1957–67.
54. Sengstaken RW, Blakemore AH. Balloon tamponage for the control of hemorrhage from esophageal varices. Ann Surg 1950;131(5):781–9.
55. Nadler J, Stankovic N, Uber A, et al. Outcomes in variceal hemorrhage following the use of a balloon tamponade device. Am J Emerg Med 2017;35(10):1500–2.
56. Choi JY, Jo YW, Lee SS, et al. Outcomes of patients treated with Sengstaken-Blakemore tube for uncontrolled variceal hemorrhage. Korean J Intern Med 2018;33(4):696–704.
57. Ortiz AM, Garcia CJ, Othman MO, et al. Innovative technique for endoscopic placement of sengstaken-Blakemore tube. South Med J 2018;111(5):307–11.
58. Shao XD, Qi XS, Guo XZ. Esophageal stent for refractory variceal bleeding: a systemic review and meta-analysis. Biomed Res Int 2016;2016:4054513.
59. McCarty TR, Njei B. Self-expanding metal stents for acute refractory esophageal variceal bleeding: a systematic review and meta-analysis. Dig Endosc 2016; 28(5):539–47.
60. Pfisterer N, Riedl F, Pachofszky T, et al. Outcomes after placement of a SX-ELLA oesophageal stent for refractory variceal bleeding-A national multicentre study. Liver Int 2019;39(2):290–8.
61. Rodrigues SG, Cárdenas A, Escorsell À, et al. Balloon tamponade and esophageal stenting for esophageal variceal bleeding in cirrhosis: a systematic review and meta-analysis. Semin Liver Dis 2019;39(2):178–94.
62. Laine L. Deflating balloon tamponade: should we expand the use of stents for severe refractory esophageal variceal bleeding? Hepatology 2016;63(6):1768–70.
63. García-Pagán JC, Caca K, Bureau C, et al. Early use of TIPS in patients with cirrhosis and variceal bleeding. N Engl J Med 2010;362(25):2370–9.

Endoscopic Treatment of Gastric and Ectopic Varices

Roberto Oleas, MD, Carlos Robles-Medranda, MD*

KEYWORDS

- Gastric varix • Gastric varices • Gastrointestinal hemorrhage • Cyanoacrylates
- Endoscopic ultrasonography

KEY POINTS

- Patients with gastric varices have a 20% mortality following an initial bleeding episode.
- A high rebleeding rate and adverse events following cyanoacrylate glue injection are the 2 mains concerns of endoscopic therapy.
- Endoscopic ultrasound-guided endovascular therapies have been proposed as safer and more effective alternatives for treating gastric varices.

INTRODUCTION

Gastric variceal bleeding in patients with chronic liver disease is associated with a high mortality, which can reach as high as 20% in the 6 weeks after the index bleeding event. Moreover, the rebleeding of gastric varices is a relatively more challenging clinical scenario, with fewer therapeutic alternatives.[1,2]

Achieving the obliteration of gastric varices either before or after a bleeding episode has been one of the primary goals of clinicians, endoscopists, hepatologists, and radiologists. Medical interventions aimed at reducing portal pressure alone do not effectively achieve varix obliteration or prevent varix bleeding.[3] Current clinical guidelines endorse endoscopic treatment with glue injections as the initial treatment of choice for actively bleeding gastric varices. However, low obliteration rates and high rebleeding rates remain pitfalls of this therapy.[4–6] Initially, interventional radiologists obliterated varices with embolization coils and glue injections under fluoroscopic guidance, and transjugular intrahepatic portosystemic shunt (TIPS) was a salvage therapy.[7] Nevertheless, in recent years, the advancements in endoscopic ultrasound (EUS)-guided endovascular therapies have enabled endosonographers to implement novel interventions. Within the present narrative review, the authors summarize currently available

Funding: none.
Instituto Ecuatoriano de Enfermedades Digestivas, Torre Vitalis I, Mezzanine 3, Av. Abel Romeo S/N y Av. Juan Tanca Marengo, Guayaquil 090505, Ecuador
* Corresponding author.
E-mail address: carlosoakm@yahoo.es

1089-3261/22/© 2021 Elsevier Inc. All rights reserved.

endoscopic treatments of gastric varices and discuss the role of innovative, cutting-edge EUS-guided endovascular therapies in patients with chronic liver disease.

Gastric Varices

The development of gastric varices may be related to portal hypertension secondary to cirrhosis; however, they can also develop in the absence of portal hypertension.[2] Endoscopically, gastric varices can be classified by their location in the stomach and whether they involve the esophagus, as described by Sarin and colleagues.[2] Gastroesophageal varices type I (GOV-I), which are the most common type, arise from the lesser gastric curvature and extend to the esophagus above the gastro-esophageal junction. GOV-II appear from the gastric fundus and extend to the esophagus, similar to GOV-I. In contrast, isolated gastric varices (IGV) can be classified as IGV-I if they solely involve the gastric fundus; meanwhile, IGV-2 are defined as those that appear elsewhere in the stomach, such as in the gastric body or antrum.

Gastrointestinal bleeding remains the leading cause of death in cirrhotic patients and has been a focus of clinical research in recent years.[1] Patients with chronic liver disease in whom gastric varices develop secondary to portal hypertension have the highest mortality. Moreover, these varices bleed at lower portal pressure gradients than esophageal varices.[8] Indeed, patients with gastric varices have an annual bleeding rate of 5% to 15%.[1] Unfortunately, this life-threatening complication is associated with morbidity, mortality, rebleeding, reintervention, unexpected readmission, and decompensation in patients with chronic liver disease.

ENDOSCOPIC THERAPY FOR GASTRIC VARICES

Patients with portal hypertension have a lower prevalence of gastric varices than esophageal varices; the former bleed more severely and are associated with higher mortality.[9] Actively bleeding gastric varices require urgent implementation of safe and effective therapy, as 30% to 40% can rebleed within the first 5 days.[9] Historically, endoscopic therapy has been the mainstay treatment for gastric varices. Endoscopic band ligation and sclerotherapy were initially proposed as therapies; however, band ligation had higher rebleeding rate and lower hemostasis rate than endoscopic glue injection.[10,11] Therefore, endoscopic glue injection has become the standard and most widely available endoscopic therapy for the treatment of gastric varices, as stated in the latest Baveno VI consensus.[4]

Endoscopic Therapy with Cyanoacrylate Glue Injection

Cyanoacrylate (N-butyl-2-cyanoacrylate) is an adhesive glue that causes blood clotting when injected, which stops variceal bleeding. Cyanoacrylate is injected at a 1:1 ratio with lipiodol into the varix without protocolized dosing; however, most endoscopists inject between 0.5 mL and 1 mL in each injection (**Fig. 1**). Nevertheless, case series and reports of unexpected adverse events have been reported, namely, pulmonary or systemic glue embolism, bleeding ulcers of the injection site, peritonitis, needle impaction, and death.[12-15]

Even though glue injection is performed under direct endoscopic view, the pooled obliteration rate for this therapy was 62.6% in a recent meta-analysis of 28 cohorts and 3467 patients, which was significantly more inferior than the rates achieved with novel EUS-guided endovascular therapies. Although there was no statistically significant difference, trends toward high rates of recurrence of gastric varices and late rebleeding were noted in patients treated with endoscopic glue injection.[6]

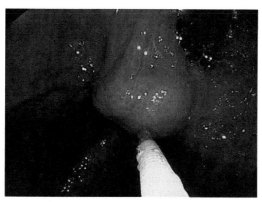

Fig. 1. Endoscopic cyanoacrylate glue injection in a patient with gastroesophageal gastric varices. (*Courtesy of* Instituto Ecuatoriano de Enfermedades Digestivas, Endoscopy Division.)

Endoscopic cyanoacrylate glue injection was compared with other endoscopic therapies in a recent meta-analysis of 6 randomized clinical trials, including only patients with chronic liver disease.[11] This study suggested that endoscopic therapy using cyanoacrylate may be more effective than endoscopic band ligation for the prevention of rebleeding from gastric varices over the course of a mean follow-up duration of 7 days (relative risk 0.60; 95% confidence interval [CI] 0.41–0.88). In addition, they found no significant differences between the 0.5-mL and 1-mL injections of glue in terms of all-cause mortality, control of bleeding, and prevention of rebleeding; however, fewer adverse events were noted in the lower-dose cyanoacrylate group.[16] In addition, this meta-analysis assessed the efficacy with regard to the control of bleeding between cyanoacrylate glue and alcohol-based compounds used for the sclerotherapy of fundal gastric varices. They found no significant differences in the control of bleeding and adverse events; however, this outcome should be corroborated by additional high-quality and well-designed studies.[17]

The considerable frequency of early and late rebleeding and the reported adverse events following endoscopic cyanoacrylate glue injection prompted interest in the identification of novel therapeutic approaches. EUS-guided therapies have been proposed as salvage interventions after failed endoscopic treatment of gastric varices.

Endoscopic primary and secondary prophylaxis of gastric varices

Even though gastric varices are found less frequently than esophageal varices in patients with chronic liver disease, an acute bleeding episode constitutes an emergency that is challenging to manage. Gastric varices greater than 20 mm, a Model for End-Stage Liver Disease score ≥ 17, and portal hypertensive gastropathy were shown to predict a severe first bleeding episode necessitating therapeutic intervention. Endoscopic cyanoacrylate therapy was compared with beta-blocker treatment and no treatment in a randomized trial, including patients with GOV-II and IGV-1, and the findings confirmed that primary endoscopic therapy is superior in preventing bleeding from gastric varices (13% of patients treated with cyanoacrylate injection had bleeding from gastric varices vs 28% of those treated with beta-blockers vs 45% of those that received no treatment, $P = .003$), improving the probability of survival over a median follow-up duration of 26 months.[18]

The prevention of a rebleeding episode following an acute bleeding episode by beta-blocker therapy and endoscopic cyanoacrylate therapy was compared in a randomized controlled trial. The gastric variceal rebleeding rate was significantly lower in patients treated endoscopically, whereas 55% of the patients treated with medical treatment experienced rebleeding.[19]

Endoscopic Therapy with thrombin Injection

Endoscopic therapy with cyanoacrylate glue injection is the most widely available option for the endoscopic treatment of bleeding gastric varices; however, bleeding ulcers at the injection site and systemic embolisms are the main disadvantages of this technique, and reports of damage to the endoscopic equipment should not be ignored.[20] Thrombin has been proposed as an alternative to glue injection. Thrombin enhances the coagulation cascade by converting fibrinogen into fibrin and enhancing platelet aggregation. It has been shown to result in hemostasis without the inducement of ulcers or nonfatal and fatal embolic complications, as observed with cyanoacrylate glue. A recent randomized trial compared these 2 endoscopic techniques and reported similar outcomes in terms of the achievement of hemostasis in patients with actively bleeding gastric varices and early and late rebleeding rates. Nevertheless, injection-induced gastric ulcers ranging from 5 to 20 mm were noted in 36.7% of the patients treated with cyanoacrylate glue, whereas none of the patients in the thrombin group developed ulcers. In addition, a higher incidence of adverse events was noted in the cyanoacrylate glue group (51.4% vs 12.1%; $P<.001$).[21]

A recent meta-analysis of 11 studies found pooled early and late rebleeding rates of 9.3% and 13.8%, respectively, suggesting that thrombin injection and endoscopic glue injection were comparable in this regard. One of the most exciting findings was the low pooled adverse event rate after the injection of thrombin into actively bleeding gastric varices (5.6%).[22] This low adverse event rate underscores the safety profile of this promising endoscopic alternative. The comparable hemostasis and early and late rebleeding rates in the randomized trial indicated that thrombin injection has a similar efficacy to that of cyanoacrylate glue.

ENDOSCOPIC ULTRASOUND-GUIDED TREATMENT OF GASTRIC VARICES
Rationale for Endoscopic Ultrasound-Guided Endovascular Therapy

Several studies have compared conventional endoscopic glue injection with novel EUS-guided endovascular therapy with either glue injection, coils, or combined coils and glue injection. Two main factors have supported the rationale for EUS-guided treatment: the efficacy of endoscopic therapy as indicated by the obliteration rate and rebleeding recurrence rate and the safety as indicated by the overall distal embolization rate.

Furthermore, there are also technical aspects that support the use of the novel EUS-guided endovascular approach. First, endoscopic ultrasonography permits direct visualization and evaluation of the gastric varix itself, which may translate into a safer glue injection because of the imaging-directed approach. Second, the EUS console allows Doppler assessment of the variceal blood flow, which enables confirmation of varix obliteration within the same treatment session.

Recently, endosonographers have implemented endosonographic varicealography in clinical practice (**Fig. 2**). This EUS-guided evaluation of gastric varices under radiologic evaluation following contrast media injection offers several pieces of information that can be used to determine the most appropriate therapeutic approach. First, it allows the assessment of the anatomy near the gastric varices, preventing the inadvertent embolization of the splenic vein, which could exacerbate portal hypertension. Indeed, endosonographic varicealography enables the classification of gastric varices into localized and diffuse gastric varices[23] and the flow trajectory as either afferent or

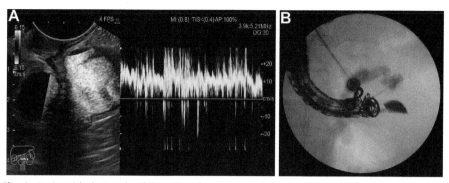

Fig. 2. EUS-guided Doppler (*A*) and endosonographic varicealography (*B*) evaluation in a patient with rebleeding gastric varices refractory to EUS-guided coil embolization. (*Courtesy of* Instituto Ecuatoriano de Enfermedades Digestivas, Endoscopy Division.)

efferent. Following EUS-guided fine-needle puncture and injection of varix, endosonographers can confirm the feeder vessel to the gastric varix and decide whether to inject cyanoacrylate glue or perform embolization at this point. This modification to the original technique was proposed in the authors' first report, which showed excellent technical and clinical success.[24] In addition, portosystemic shunts can be detected during EUS-guided varicealography, a condition that precludes cyanoacrylate injection owing to an increased risk of systemic glue embolization, providing information that is relevant for clinical decision making.[25] Finally, this technique can be used to confirm the complete obliteration and absence of flow at the end of the procedure (**Fig. 3**).

Safety is one of the main concerns driving the shift from endoscopic to EUS-guided endovascular therapies. Regarding safety, less cyanoacrylate glue is needed to

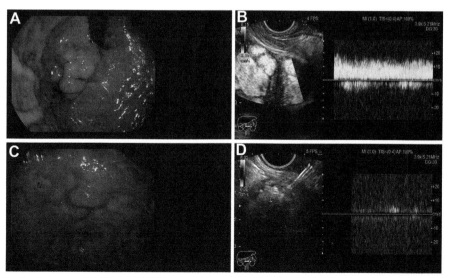

Fig. 3. Endoscopic (*A*) and EUS-Doppler (*B*) evaluation of a patient with GOV-II. Following EUS-guided combined coil embolization with cyanoacrylate injection, the authors confirmed complete obliteration under endoscopic (*C*) and endosonographic Doppler (*D*). (*Courtesy of* Instituto Ecuatoriano de Enfermedades Digestivas, Endoscopy Division.)

achieve obliteration when treating the gastric varix afferent feeder vessels.[26] Next, the authors review the available data regarding the use of EUS-guided endovascular therapies to obliterate bleeding and recently bleeding gastric varices.

Endoscopic Ultrasound-Guided Glue Injection

This endosonographic technique was originally reported by Romero-Castro and colleagues,[27] who injected cyanoacrylate glue into the afferent vessels of gastric varices. The investigators described how this EUS-guided endovascular technique offered several advantages over the endoscopic approach. The main advantages were the identification of the varices and direction of the obliterating agent under endosonographic guidance and ability to confirm the absence of flow after treatment under EUS-Doppler guidance.

Two cyanoacrylate-derivate glues have been used for this endovascular therapy: 2-octyl-cyanoacrylate, which is a relatively less dense solution that has a longer polymerization time and therefore a longer injection time that prevents glue impaction within the needle, injection site, or echoendoscope working channel, and N-butyl-cyanoacrylate, which is diluted with Lipiodol for the fluoroscopic evaluation and detection of distal glue embolisms but is a more viscous solution and therefore more challenging to inject within vessels.

A recently published study compared the endoscopic versus EUS-guided injection of 2-octyl-cyanoacrylate. Even though no difference regarding safety was reported, a significant superiority of EUS-guided cyanoacrylate glue was noted in terms of rebleeding (8.8% vs 23.7%, $P = .04$) and the number of varices injected (1.6 vs 1.1, $P<.001$); more importantly, the investigators reported that a lower mean quantity of glue was required to achieve obliteration during the index endoscopy (2 mL vs 3.3 mL, $P<.001$).[28]

Endoscopic Ultrasound-Guided Coiling

The idea of deploying embolization coils within the afferent vessels of gastric varices has been one of the latest developments in EUS-guided endovascular therapy. These embolization coils act as a mesh that induces platelet aggregation and further obstructs the flow within the feeder vessel, resulting in the complete obliteration of the varices.[29] In addition, when the coils are sized appropriately, that is, when they are larger than 120% of the varix diameter, the risk of migration is minimized. However, adverse events, such as perforation, bleeding, and coil extrusion, can occur.

EUS-guided coiling was compared against EUS-guided cyanoacrylate injection in a retrospective study. Even though there was no difference in clinical efficacy, as defined by the obliteration rate, coiling was associated with a lower adverse event rate, whereas glue injection was associated with a high incidence of asymptomatic glue embolism.[26] In addition, complete obliteration within 1 session of coiling was achieved in 82% of the patients; however, both techniques achieved similar overall obliteration rates. Twenty-five percent of patients with gastric varices may have portosystemic shunts, such as gastrorenal shunts, which is a condition that is associated with a high risk of systemic embolization when cyanoacrylate glue is injected alone; therefore, these patients may benefit from coiling therapy without the injection of cyanoacrylate glue.[25,30]

Endoscopic Ultrasound-Guided Combined Therapy

In one of the most recent meta-analyses including data on all EUS-guided endovascular modalities and endoscopic glue as a comparator, a subanalysis of data from 6 cohort studies showed that EUS-guided combined therapy was associated with a significantly lower recurrence rate of gastric varices: 5.2%, compared with 15% for EUS-guided glue injection and 18% for endoscopic glue therapy ($P = .01$).[6] This same meta-analysis demonstrated the superiority of EUS-guided endovascular treatment for obliteration of gastric varices (84.4% vs 62.6%, $P = .02$). Even though the result was not statistically significant, trends toward better outcomes in terms of treatment efficacy and the prevention of early and late rebleeding were noted for all EUS-guided modalities.[6]

EUS-guided combined therapy was compared against coiling alone in a randomized controlled trial involving 60 patients. Both techniques showed excellent technical success and obliteration rates. However, combined treatment was associated with a lower incidence of rebleeding (20% vs 3.3%, $P = .04$). Moreover, this group of patients was more likely to not need reintervention (hazard ratio 0.27; 95% CI 0.09–0.79; $P = .01$). Interestingly, in a subanalysis excluding patients treated for primary prophylaxis, coiling alone was associated with significantly higher rebleeding, gastric varix reappearance, and reintervention rates. In addition, they found that actively bleeding varices treated with coiling alone were particularly likely to reappear during follow-up.[31]

Another meta-analysis including data on 3 EUS-guided endovascular therapies, namely, EUS-guided cyanoacrylate injection, EUS-guided coiling alone, and EUS-guided combined therapy with coil embolization and cyanoacrylate injection, showed that the latest exhibited better technical and clinical success than EUS-guided cyanoacrylate injection (100% vs 97%, $P<.001$ and 98% vs 96%, $P<.001$, respectively). In addition, they reported a lower adverse event rate for EUS-guided combined therapy than for EUS-guided cyanoacrylate glue injection (10% vs 21%, $P<01$), whereas similar adverse event rates were noted for EUS-guided combined therapy and EUS-guided coiling alone (10% vs 3%, $P = .06$).[32]

Primary prophylaxis of gastric variceal bleeding with EUS-guided coil and glue injection was assessed in an observational study involving 80 patients with high-risk gastric varices. During a mean follow-up duration of 3 years, only 2.5% developed bleeding from gastric varices. Moreover, emergency TIPS was not required, and no deaths related to gastric variceal bleeding were reported in this cohort.[33]

Endoscopic Ultrasound-Guided Embolization with Absorbable Hemostatic Gelatin Sponges

EUS-guided combined coil embolization and injection of hemostatic absorbable gelatin sponge was described in a recent retrospective review. This absorbable gelatin sponge converts into a liquid slurry following the deployment of the embolization coils. Excellent feasibility and safety as well as an absence of rebleeding or required reintervention were reported, with all patients who underwent follow-up EUS showing nearly total variceal obliteration.[34] Later, a matched cohort study with prospective data collection compared this novel technique with endoscopic cyanoacrylate glue injection. Both methods showed similar technical success and adverse event rates; however, EUS-guided combined coil embolization with absorbable hemostatic gelatin sponge injection showed a more prolonged time to reintervention, less rebleeding, and reduced need for blood transfusion and reintervention than endoscopic cyanoacrylate therapy.[35]

Refractory bleeding following standard cyanoacrylate glue injection

Endoscopic cyanoacrylate injection is the current standard therapy for managing bleeding gastric varices. Nevertheless, 25% to 50% of patients will experience rebleeding. Therefore, various interventions have been proposed, including EUS-guided coil embolization combined with or without cyanoacrylate injection or a second endoscopic attempt at cyanoacrylate injection. A recent retrospective study evaluated the most appropriate approach for the treatment of gastric variceal rebleeding after cyanoacrylate injection. Reintervention with EUS-guided coil embolization with or without cyanoacrylate injection was superior to a second endoscopic attempt at cyanoacrylate glue injection in terms of rebleeding (20% vs 51%, P<.001).[36]

Economic implications of endoscopic therapies for gastric varices

Gastrointestinal bleeding is not only the leading cause of death in patients with chronic liver disease but also the most expensive complication in terms of hospitalizations.[37] Originally, endoscopic treatment with cyanoacrylate glue injection was shown to be more cost-effective than TIPS for the management of bleeding gastric varices, based on the cost of the procedure itself and the length of hospitalization. Patients treated with endoscopic glue injection incurred a significantly lower median cost within 6 months of the initial gastric variceal bleeding than those treated with TIPS ($4138 vs $11,906; P<.001).[38]

Repeated endoscopic cyanoacrylate glue injection until variceal obliteration was achieved and the recently developed EUS-guided combined therapy with coil embolization and cyanoacrylate glue injection were compared in a single-center, retrospective cost-effectiveness analysis. The investigators reported that even though the EUS-guided combined therapy was more expensive, the overall cost of treatment, which included interventions for rebleeding episodes and hospitalizations, was significantly higher in the endoscopic cyanoacrylate glue treatment group.[39] Indeed, endoscopic therapy was associated with increased health-related costs of $2670, $8012, and $127 for early rebleeding, adverse events, and day of hospitalization, respectively. However, more extensive multicenter trials should be conducted to determine the real-world economic impact of EUS-guided endovascular therapies for gastric varices.

Future perspectives

Currently available data highlight the limitations of endoscopic cyanoacrylate glue injection not only in terms of feasibility during active gastric variceal bleeding but also in terms of preventing early and late rebleeding; nevertheless, this therapy is included in the current clinical guidelines and is the most widely available treatment worldwide. EUS-guided endovascular interventions have yielded promising results in terms of their clinical efficacy and safety profiles; however, these techniques require a complex training process. In addition, a limited number of endoscopic facilities offer this therapeutic alternative to patients. In the future, development of an established curriculum for EUS-guided endovascular therapy and an increase in the number of expert endosonographers worldwide should be priorities for clinical societies. In addition, the robust evidence available supports the updating of the current recommendations to include EUS-guided endovascular therapy with combined coil embolization and cyanoacrylate glue injection as the first-line therapy in those facilities that offer this procedure. Endoscopic cyanoacrylate injection should be offered only in units in which EUS-guided endovascular therapies are not available. The proposal to use thrombin injection instead of cyanoacrylate glue injection for the endoscopic treatment of gastric varices is a promising alternative that could improve the safety profile.

The authors have experienced a shift from the treatment of gastric varices with endoscopic glue injection to the use of EUS-guided endovascular interventions. Within the authors' endoscopy unit, endoscopic therapy with cyanoacrylate glue injection was associated with a 15.8% early rebleeding rate and the failure to achieve hemostasis during the index endoscopy.[39] Therefore, implementing more effective interventions was one of their main treatment goals. At this time, approximately 130 patients have been treated with an EUS-guided intervention in the authors' center, with most patients treated with combined coil embolization and cyanoacrylate glue injection, based on their recently published findings.[24,31]

SUMMARY

In conclusion, gastric variceal bleeding is a catastrophic complication of portal hypertension. Novel endoscopic and endosonographic interventions have demonstrated feasibility and clinical efficacy, ultimately resulting in decreased mortality following the index bleeding event. The current clinical guidelines fail to reflect available data, and further changes in clinical practice await implementation.

CLINICS CARE POINTS

- A gastric variceal bleeding episode has a 20% associated mortality.
- Gastric varices can rebleed in up to 30-40% of patients within the first five days.
- Endoscopic injection of cyanoacrylate glue has a 62% obliteration rate.
- Endoscopic ultrasound-guided therapy with combined coping and glue injection has a 97% clinical success and a lower adverse event rate.

AUTHOR'S CONTRIBUTIONS

R. Oleas and C. Robles-Medranda contributed equally to the conception and design of the work, drafting of the article, and critical revision for important intellectual content. Both authors approved the final version of the article to be published.

CONFLICT OF INTERESTS

R. Oleas has nothing to disclose. C. Robles-Medranda is a key opinion leader and consultant for Pentax Medical, Boston Scientific, Steris, Medtronic, Motus, Microtech, G-Tech Medical Supply, Creo Medical, and Medicons Group.

REFERENCES

1. Carbonell N, Pauwels A, Serfaty L, et al. Improved survival after variceal bleeding in patients with cirrhosis over the past two decades. Hepatology 2000;40(3):652–9.
2. Sarin SK, Lahoti D, Saxena SP, et al. Prevalence, classification and natural history of gastric varices: a long-term follow-up study in 568 portal hypertension patients. Hepatology 1992;16(6):1343–9.
3. Wu CY, Yeh HZ, Chen GH. Pharmacologic efficacy in gastric variceal rebleeding and survival: including multivariate analysis. J Clin Gastroenterol 2002;35(2): 127–32.
4. de Franchis R, Faculty BV. Expanding consensus in portal hypertension: report of the Baveno VI Consensus Workshop: stratifying risk and individualizing care for portal hypertension. J Hepatol 2015;63:743–52.
5. Guo YW, Miao HB, Wen ZF, et al. Procedure-related complications in gastric variceal obturation with tissue glue. World J Gastroenterol 2017;23(43):7746–55.

6. Mohan BP, Chandan S, Khan SR, et al. Efficacy and safety of endoscopic ultrasound-guided therapy versus direct endoscopic glue injection therapy for gastric varices: systematic review and meta-analysis. Endoscopy 2020;52:259–67.

7. Perry BC, Kwan SW. Portosystemic shunts: stable utilization and improved outcomes, two decades after the transjugular intrahepatic portosystemic shunt. J Am Coll Radiol 2015;12(12):1427–33.

8. Irani S, Kowdley K, Kozarek R. Gastric varices: an updated review of management. J Clin Gastroenterol 2011;45(2):133–48.

9. Franchis R. Upper digestive bleeding in cirrhosis. Post-therapeutic outcome and prognostic indicators. Hepatology 2003;38(3):599–612.

10. Qiao W, Ren Y, Bai Y, et al. Cyanoacrylate injection versus band ligation in the endoscopic management of acute gastric variceal bleeding: meta-analysis of randomized, controlled studies based on the PRISMA statement. Med (United States) 2015;94(41):e1725.

11. Ríos Castellanos E, Seron P, Gisbert JP, et al. Endoscopic injection of cyanoacrylate glue versus other endoscopic procedures for acute bleeding gastric varices in people with portal hypertension. Cochrane Database Syst Rev 2015;(5): CD010180.

12. Kok K, Bond RP, Duncan IC, et al. Distal embolization and local vessel wall ulceration after gastric obliteration with N-butyl-2-cyanoacrylate: a case report and review of the literature. Endoscopy 2004;36(5):442–6.

13. Bhasin D, Sharma B, Prasad H, et al. Endoscopic removal of sclerotherapy needle from gastric varix after N-butyl-2-cyanoacrylate injection. Gastrointest Endosc 2000;51:497–8.

14. Saracco G, Giordanino C, Roberto N, et al. Fatal multiple systemic embolisms after injection of cyanoacrylate in bleeding gastric varices of a patient who was noncirrhotic but with idiopathic portal hypertension. Gastrointest Endosc 2007; 65:345–7.

15. Rickman O, Utz J, Aughenbaugh G, et al. Pulmonary embolization of 2-octyl cyanoacrylate after endoscopic injection therapy for gastric variceal bleeding. Mayo Clin Proc 2004;79:1455–8.

16. Hou MC, Lin HC, Lee HS, et al. A randomized trial of endoscopic cyanoacrylate injection for acute gastric variceal bleeding: 0.5 mL versus 1.0 mL. Gastrointest Endosc 2009;70(4):668–75.

17. Sarin SK, Jain AK, Jain M, et al. A randomized controlled trial of cyanoacrylate versus alcohol injection in patients with isolated fundic varices. Am J Gastroenterol 2002;97(4):1010–5.

18. Mishra SR, Sharma BC, Kumar A, et al. Primary prophylaxis of gastric variceal bleeding comparing cyanoacrylate injection and beta-blockers: a randomized controlled trial. J Hepatol 2011;54(6):1161–7.

19. Mishra SR, Sharma BC, Kumar A, et al. Endoscopic cyanoacrylate injection versus β-blocker for secondary prophylaxis of gastric variceal bleed: a randomized controlled trial. Gut 2010;59(6):729–35.

20. Tripathi D, Ferguson JW, Therapondos G, et al. Review article: recent advances in the management of bleeding gastric varices. Aliment Pharmacol Ther 2006; 24:1–17.

21. Lo GH, Lin CW, Tai CM, et al. A prospective, randomized trial of thrombin versus cyanoacrylate injection in the control of acute gastric variceal hemorrhage. Endoscopy 2020;52(7):548–55.

22. Bhurwal A, Makar M, Patel A, et al. Safety and efficacy of thrombin for bleeding gastric varices: a systematic review and meta-analysis. Dig Dis Sci 2021. [Epub ahead of print].

23. Arakawa M, Masuzaki T, Okuda K. Pathology of fundic varices of the stomach and rupture. J Gastroenterol Hepatol 2002;17(10):1064–9.

24. Robles-Medranda C, Valero M, Nebel JA, et al. Endoscopic-ultrasound-guided coil and cyanoacrylate embolization for gastric varices and the roles of endoscopic Doppler and endosonographic varicealography in vascular targeting. Dig Endosc 2019;31(3):283–90.

25. Wang XM, Yu S, Chen X, et al. Endoscopic ultrasound-guided injection of coils and cyanoacrylate glue for the treatment of gastric fundal varices with abnormal shunts: a series of case reports. J Int Med Res 2019;47(4):1802–9.

26. Romero-Castro R, Ellrichmann M, Ortiz-Moyano C, et al. EUS-guided coil versus cyanoacrylate therapy for the treatment of gastric varices: a multicenter study (with videos). Gastrointest Endosc 2013;78(5):711–21.

27. Romero-Castro R, Pellicer-Bautista FJ, Jimenez-Saenz M, et al. EUS-guided injection of cyanoacrylate in perforating feeding veins in gastric varices: results in 5 cases. Gastrointest Endosc 2007;66(2):402–7.

28. Bick B, Al-Haddad M, Liangpunsakul S, et al. EUS-guided fine needle injection is superior to direct endoscopic injection of 2-octyl cyanoacrylate for the treatment of gastric variceal bleeding. Surg Endosc 2018;33(6):1837–45.

29. Romero-Castro R, Pellicer-Bautista F, Giovannini M, et al. Endoscopic ultrasound (EUS)-guided coil embolization therapy in gastric varices. Endoscopy 2010;42(S 02):E35–6.

30. Kakutani H, Hino S, Ikeda K, et al. Use of the curved linear-array echo endoscope to identify gastrorenal shunts in patients with gastric fundal varices. Endoscopy 2004;36(8):710–4.

31. Robles-Medranda C, Oleas R, Valero M, et al. Endoscopic ultrasonography-guided deployment of embolization coils and cyanoacrylate injection in gastric varices versus coiling alone: a randomized trial. Endoscopy 2020;52(4):268–75.

32. McCarty T, Bazarbashi A, Hathorn K, et al. Combination therapy versus monotherapy for EUS-guided management of gastric varices: a systematic review and meta-analysis. Endosc Ultrasound 2019;9(1):6–15.

33. Kouanda A, Binmoeller K, Hamerski C, et al. Safety and efficacy of EUS-guided coil and glue injection for the primary prophylaxis of gastric variceal hemorrhage. Gastrointest Endosc 2021;94(2):291–6.

34. Bazarbashi AN, Wang TJ, Thompson CC, et al. Endoscopic ultrasound-guided treatment of gastric varices with coil embolization and absorbable hemostatic gelatin sponge: a novel alternative to cyanoacrylate. Endosc Int Open 2020; 08(02):E221–7.

35. Bazarbashi AN, Wang TJ, Jirapinyo P, et al. Endoscopic ultrasound-guided coil embolization with absorbable gelatin sponge appears superior to traditional cyanoacrylate injection for the treatment of gastric varices. Clin Transl Gastroenterol 2020;11(5):e00175.

36. Mukkada RJ, Antony R, Chooracken MJ, et al. Endoscopic ultrasound-guided coil or glue injection in post-cyanoacrylate gastric variceal rebleed. Indian J Gastroenterol 2018;37(2):153–9.

37. Talwalkar JA. Cost-effectiveness of treating esophageal varices. Clin Liver Dis 2006;10:679–89.

38. Mahadeva S, Bellamy MC, Kessel D, et al. Cost-effectiveness of N-butyl-2-cyanoacrylate (histoacryl) glue injections versus transjugular intrahepatic

portosystemic shunt in the management of acute gastric variceal bleeding. Am J Gastroenterol 2003;98:2688–93.

39. Robles-Medranda C, Nebel JA, Puga-Tejada M, et al. Cost-effectiveness of endoscopic ultrasound-guided coils plus cyanoacrylate injection compared to endoscopic cyanoacrylate injection in the management of gastric varices. World J Gastrointest Endosc 2021;13(1):13–23.

Role of Endoscopic Retrograde Cholangiopancreatography in the Diagnosis and Management of Cholestatic Liver Diseases

Tara Keihanian, MD, MPH[a], Monique T. Barakat, MD, PhD[b],
Sooraj Tejaswi, MD, MSPH[c], Rajnish Mishra, MD[d],
Christopher J. Carlson, MD[d], John J. Brandabur, MD[d],
Mohit Girotra, MD[d],*

KEYWORDS

- Endoscopic retrograde cholangiopancreatography • ERCP
- Cholestatic liver diseases • Primary sclerosing cholangitis • PSC
- Autoimmune cholangiopathy • Postliver transplant stricture
- Infectious associated cholangiopathy

INTRODUCTION

Cholestatic liver diseases (CLDs) entail a variety of diseases involving the bile ducts, intrahepatic or extrahepatic, or combination of both, resulting from primary and secondary bile duct injuries.[1] Among the most common causes of CLDs are primary sclerosing cholangitis (PSC), primary biliary cholangitis (PBC), and medication-induced liver injury. There is an exhaustive list of medications known to cause cholestatic hepatic panel, including but not limited to oral contraceptives, anabolic steroids, estrogens, anticonvulsants [phenytoin, carbamazepine, and so forth.], cyclosporin, azathioprine, chemotherapy agents such as 5-flourouracile, dapsone, and antibiotics [erythromycin, nitrofurantoin, amoxicillin–clavulanic acid, and so forth].[1] Total parenteral nutrition (TPN) is also known to results in cholestatic liver injury in long-term users. Henceforth, to develop an accurate differential diagnosis of CLDs, obtaining a thorough medical, surgical, and drug/medication history is of utmost importance.

[a] Division of Gastroenterology, Baylor College of Medicine, 7200 Cambridge Street, Suite A8, Houston, TX 77030, USA; [b] Division of Gastroenterology, Stanford University School of Medicine, 300 Pasteur Drive # 5244, Stanford, CA 94304, USA; [c] Division of Gastroenterology, Sutter Medical Group, 2068 John Jones Road, Davis, CA 95161, USA; [d] Digestive Health Institute, Swedish Medical Center, 1221 Madison Street, Arnold Pavilion, Suite 1220, Seattle, WA 98104, USA
* Corresponding author.
E-mail address: Mohit.Girotra@Swedish.org

Clin Liver Dis 26 (2022) 51–67
https://doi.org/10.1016/j.cld.2021.08.006
1089-3261/22/© 2021 Elsevier Inc. All rights reserved.

liver.theclinics.com

The most common cause of extrahepatic biliary obstruction is choledocholithiasis. Other etiologies of extrahepatic biliary obstruction include benign or malignant biliary stricture/obstruction, autoimmune diseases [immunoglobulin G (IgG)-4 related cholangiopathy], malformations, and infections. Malignant obstructions can be due to pancreatic cancer, gallbladder cancer, ampullary cancer, cholangiocarcinoma (CCA), and perihilar lymph nodes with external compression over the biliary system (lymphoma vs metastatic). Other biliary strictures could result from prior complicated endoscopic or surgical procedures, chronic pancreatitis, and posttransplant. Common infections known to cause extrahepatic duct injury include acquired immunodeficiency syndrome cholangiopathy (AIDS cholangiopathy), *Ascaris lumbricoides,* and liver flukes. On the other hand, intrahepatic cholestasis can be due to toxins and/or medications (as previously mentioned), immune-mediated etiologies (which include PSC, PBC), and infiltrative diseases such as amyloidosis, sarcoidosis, and tuberculosis. Other less common causes may be alcohol-associated hepatitis, ischemic cholangiopathy (IsC), liver allograft rejection, sickle cell disease, and intrahepatic cholestasis of pregnancy (ICP).[1]

The initial approach to establish a diagnosis of CLDs includes obtaining proper serologic workup, followed by abdominal ultrasound (US), computed tomography (CT) scan, or magnetic resonance imaging and cholangiopancreatography (MRI/MRCP) as the preferred imaging modalities. The role of endoscopic retrograde cholangiopancreatography (ERCP) as an initial diagnostic modality for CLDs is limited, and considering advances in radiological imaging in the last few decades have enabled high-quality assessment; however, ERCP is uniquely advantageous in that it enables tissue sampling for diagnosis and further genetic and molecular testing, and stent placement to relieve the biliary obstruction. The main focus of our review article is to appraise the role of ERCP in diagnosis and management in the variety of CLDs.

Primary sclerosing cholangitis

PSC is a progressive chronic CLDs resulting in multifocal biliary duct stenosis and strictures, which may develop at any level of the biliary tree, from microscopic intrahepatic biliary radicles to large extrahepatic biliary ducts. Although PSC usually involves both intrahepatic and extrahepatic bile ducts, it may be localized to intrahepatic and extrahepatic bile ducts in 11% and 2% of cases, respectively.[2] MRCP is the preferred first step in the diagnostic algorithm, given its noninvasive nature and ability to provide adequate radiological information to establish the diagnosis firmly. The typical cholangiographic appearance of PSC includes "beaded" appearance of bile ducts and diffuse, multifocal, and circumferential strictures alternating with normal or minimally dilated duct in between,[2,3] which can be well visualized on MRCP (**Fig. 1**). However, limitations of MRCP include low sensitivity for identifying subtle early changes in intrahepatic PSC and limited accuracy in the differentiation of PSC from secondary sclerosing cholangitis (SSC), thus ERCP has remained the gold standard for the diagnosis of early PSC in certain patient populations.[4] Due to impaired biliary flow and bacterial overgrowth in patients with PSC who have dominant stricture (DS), there is a higher risk of upstream stone formation, symptomatic choledocholithiasis, and cholangitis, warranting endoscopic therapy to relieve the obstruction, which is an additional benefit ERCP has over diagnostic MRCP.

Dominant stricture in primary sclerosing cholangitis

A DS is usually suspected in patients with PSC with new signs/symptoms of biliary obstruction and/or worsening cholestasis. Chronic biliary obstruction due to DS could potentially lead to accelerated hepatic fibrosis and cirrhosis, and reversal of this

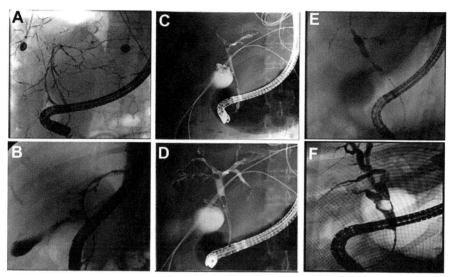

Fig. 1. ERCP representation of PSC findings – (*A*): diffuse intrahepatic PSC disease (beaded appearance with diffuse multifocal circumferential strictures with normal or minimally dilated ducts in between); (*B*): dominant stricture (DS) in the right main hepatic duct (R-IHD); (*C*): DS in the common hepatic duct (CHD) and left main hepatic duct (LIHD); (*D*): DS in the common bile duct (CBD) with upstream biliary sludge/casts; (*E*): DS in CHD and extensive intrahepatic duct (IHD) disease; (*F*): DS in distal CBD with upstream choledocholithiasis.

cholestatic injury may be achieved by relieving the biliary obstruction.[5] A DS is typically encountered in 36% to 50% of patients with PSC over time,[2] and the appropriate first step in such a scenario is noninvasive imaging such as MRI/MRCP or a contrast-enhanced CT. Long, rapidly evolving, or very tight strictures should increase suspicion for CCA and warrant dedicated evaluation with ERCP for ductal sampling by brush cytology and/or endobiliary tissue acquisition for histopathological evaluation.[2] DS is defined as a stenosis diameter measuring less than 1.5 mm in the extrahepatic duct or less than 1.0 mm in the intrahepatic duct[6] (see **Fig. 1**B–E), and differentiating benign from malignant DS is challenging. Patients with DS tend to have poor long-term outcome, secondary to a higher risk of CCA or cholestasis and progressive fibrosis leading to cirrhosis. A 25-year longitudinal single-center experience from United Kingdom on 128 patients with PSC suggested worse survival in patients with DS (mean 13.7 years vs 23 years without DS), with much of survival difference attributable to 26% risk of CCA in patients with DS, with half of those CCA presenting within 4 months of diagnosis of DS, thus underscoring the importance of an exhaustive evaluation of a new DS.[7]

Brush cytology historically has been the initial diagnostic modality of choice to appraise the nature of DS, albeit hampered by low sensitivity. A recent meta-analysis (11 studies, 747 patients) showed pooled 43% sensitivity (95% confidence interval (CI): 35–52) and 97% specificity of bile duct brushings for a diagnosis of CCA in PSC.[8] In fact, the literature reports a wide range of accuracy (8%–85%) of bile duct brushing for the diagnosis of CCA in PSC,[9,10] with these observed discrepancies attributable to tumor size and/or location making adequate tissue sampling challenging, and additionally pathologic diagnostic limitations owing to acellular tissue due to the desmoplastic nature of the DS.[8] It is hence recommended that patients with negative or atypical brush cytology results should undergo close ongoing monitoring. In 2013, Witt *and colleagues* proposed a weighted scoring system called atypical biliary brushing score (ABBS) to assist risk-stratifying patients with atypical strictures.[11] The score consisted of 7 variables (1 point for age >60, procedure indication of pancreatic mass, stricture in the distal common bile duct, CA 19-9 > 300 U/mL; 2 points for the endoscopic impression of malignancy, common hepatic duct stricture, and the presence of PSC),[11] and a score ≥4 was considered at greater risk for malignancy; however, this scoring system was never validated.[11]

The poor sensitivity of conventional brush cytology alone has encouraged the emergence of newer techniques to enhance diagnostic yield. The most important additive technique is fluorescence in situ hybridization (FISH), which increases sensitivity to 64%, and positive predictive value to 69% in presence of polysomy on 2 sequential specimens.[12] In a study from the Mayo Clinic of 235 PSC patients with DS, 120 (51%) tested positive for FISH, but 1/3 (35/120) of those had confirmed CCA on histopathological evaluation.[13] The authors inferred that in patients with PSC, the presence of DS plus FISH polysomy confers 88% specificity for CCA (although sensitivity was still low at 46%), whereas FISH trisomy/tetrasomy performed relatively lower (sensitivity 25%, specificity 67%).[13] In a subsequent meta-analysis (8 studies, 828 patients), the pooled sensitivity and specificity of FISH for the diagnosis of CCA in patients with PSC were 68% (95% CI: 61–74) and 70% (95% CI: 66–73), respectively, whereas the respective numbers for FISH polysomy (6 studies, 690 patients) were 51% and 93%.[14] These data support high specificity (88%–93%) of FISH polysomy for CCA diagnosis in patients with PSC, but due to low sensitivity (46%–51%), further research is ongoing.[13,14] With advances in next-generation sequencing (NGS) for cancer diagnosis, a combination of 28-gene NGS panel (BiliSeq) and pathologic evaluation yielded 83% sensitivity and 99% specificity for the diagnosis of malignant stricture in patients with PSC.[15] BiliSeq improved the sensitivity of biliary brushings for the diagnosis of malignancy from 35% to 77% and biliary biopsies from 52% to 83%.[15]

A major game-changing advancement in the diagnosis of indeterminate biliary strictures occurred with the introduction of single operator cholangioscope (SOC) (SpyGlass Direct Visualization System [Boston Scientific, Marlborough, MA, USA]), which allows for the direct examination of the biliary tract mucosa and vascular pattern (**Fig. 2**). This modality also enables the acquisition of a bile duct epithelium directly from the abnormal tissue site using SpyBite biopsy forceps (Boston Scientific, Marlborough, MA, USA). This platform also provides additional therapeutic benefits including stone lithotripsy and tissue ablation.[16] A meta-analysis in 2016 involving 21 studies showed that all other ERCP-based interventions (cytology, FISH, confocal laser endomicroscopy), ERCP cholangioscopy with targeted biopsies was the most accurate (96%; 95% CI: 94–97) modality for diagnosing CCA in patients with PSC, with pooled sensitivity and specificity being 65% and 97%, respectively.[17] According to a prospective Swedish study of 47 patients with PSC, cholangioscopy alone failed to distinguish between benign and malignant strictures.[18] Using narrow-band imaging (NBI) during cholangioscopy allowed a 48% increase in suspicious lesions biopsied with NBI compared with white light and also allowed better visualization of tumor margins, although NBI directed biopsies did not improve the dysplasia detection rate.[19] Although cholangioscopy definitely opened a new horizon in the diagnosis and management of DS in patients with PSC, its larger outer diameter (~10Fr) usually requires endoscopic sphincterotomy or sphincteroplasty as well as stricture dilation to be able to pass the device to target stricture for biopsies, and may impose additional complications postprocedure.[20] Majeed and colleagues in their study of 225 patients with PSC undergoing liver transplantation (LT) noted highest sensitivity for the detection

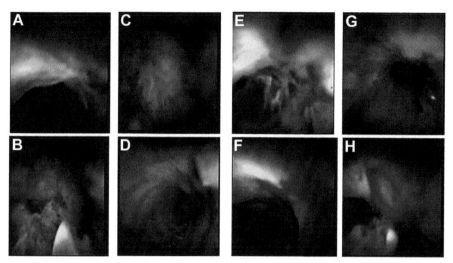

Fig. 2. Cholangioscopic representation of PSC changes/findings – (*A*): Fibrosis changes in bile duct; (*B*): hilum with upstream biliary casts; (*C*): edematous bile duct wall; (*D*): proximal CBD/CHD stricture; (*E*): proximal stricture with upstream choledocholithiasis; (*F*): distal CBD stricture; (*G*): bile duct chronic ulcer; (*H*): neovascularzation changes in CBD wall, raising early concern for CCA.

of CCA and high-grade dysplasia (HGD) with SOC directed targeted examination (100%) followed by FISH (84%), then repeated ERCP-brush cytology (82%) with modest 57% sensitivity for single ERCP-brush cytology.[21] A prospective open-label multicenter trial from France noted SOC to have a dramatic impact on the management of patients with indeterminate biliary strictures and PSC with suspected CCA, influencing decisions regarding surgical resection versus conservative management.[22]

Probe-based confocal endomicroscopy (pCLE) is another ERCP-based tool with an evolving and promising role in the investigation of patients with DS with PSC. A recent prospective multicenter US-based study from 2021 used pCLE for the evaluation of 63 strictures in 59 patients.[23] The overall sensitivity and specificity of pCLE were 85.7% (95% CI: 42.1–99.6) and 73.1% (95% CI: 58.9–84.4), respectively,[24] and with respect to stricture location, pCLE sensitivity was high for stricture at the bifurcation (100%) and the right hepatic duct (RHD) (100%), but low for common bile duct, common bile duct (CBD) (25%), and left hepatic duct (LHD) (28%).[24]

Management of dominant stricture

Endoscopic interventions on DS have a high yield in achieving diminished symptoms of pruritus or cholangitis, reduction of cholestasis, and measurable improvement of strictures radiologically.[23] Although not further validated, a recent French study has suggested a robust response to endoscopic therapy at 12 months in patients with PSC with pruritus and hyperbilirubinemia/transaminasemia, who have severe CBD stricture or short LHD stricture.[25] Among endoscopic therapies, biliary endoscopic balloon dilation (EBD) is generally preferred over endoscopic biliary stenting (EBS) in the management of long PSC strictures, whenever malignancy is excluded.[26] Gotthardt and colleagues in 2010 reported single-center 20-year experience of their cohort of patients with PSC (n = 171), of which 20 had DS at initiation period, and 77 more patients developed DS over time.[27] 500 serial EBD were performed over the years, with reported adverse events of pancreatitis (2.2%), bacterial cholangitis (1.4%), and bile duct perforation (0.2%), whereas only 5 patients with complete obstruction with bacterial cholangitis were stented.[27] This EBD strategy achieved a robust 5-year (81%) and 10-year (52%) survival free of LT after the first dilation of a DS.[27]

Not all DS respond adequately to serial EBD and occasionally bile duct stenting becomes inevitable. This could be due to the etiology of the stricture (**Fig. 3**). Fibrostenotic strictures (see **Fig. 3**A) may respond better to EBD than acute inflammatory narrowing (see **Fig. 3**B) of the bile ducts. Cholangioscopic classification of PSC into acute inflammation, chronic inflammation, and fibrostenotic disease (see **Fig. 3**) might help identify patients likely to respond to endoscopic interventions such as EBD or EBS.[28] A systematic review by Boeckel and colleagues (47 studies, 1116 patients with PSC with DS) showed that while technical success was high, the clinical success rates for multiple plastic stents (PSs), uncovered self-expandable metal stents, and single PS were 94.3%, 79.5%, and 59.6%, respectively.[29] However, data included in this systematic review were primarily from case series (46 out of 47 included studies), with only 1 nonrandomized comparative study, and no randomized controlled trial (RCT).[29] Stenting for a short duration of time (median = 9 days) has been shown to reduce the risk of stent occlusion and led to the reduction of cholestasis in most patients (81%).[30] However, this EBS strategy still carries a higher complication profile. According to a retrospective study of 71 patients with PSC from the Mayo Clinic by Kaya and colleagues (EBD alone = 34, EBD + EBS = 37, groups comparable at baseline in terms of age, symptoms, and bilirubin levels), the overall complication rate (30 vs 6, $P = .001$) and acute cholangitis ($P = .004$) were higher in the EBS group than the EBD only group,[31] with no significant difference in the improvement of cholestasis between the 2 groups. Moreover, percutaneous stenting had higher complication profile in comparison to EBS (23 vs 7, $P = .001$),[31] which further emphasizes the importance of the endoscopic approach as opposed to

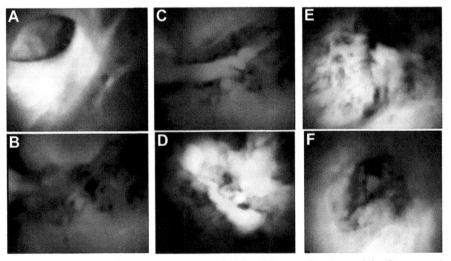

Fig. 3. Cholangioscopic features of variants of PSC and its complications – (*A*): Fibro-stenotic variant of PSC; (*B*): acute inflammatory variant of PSC; (*C*): acute purulent PSC; (*D*): CCA arising from IPMN-B; (*E*): CCA arising from distal CBD DS; (*F*): CCA arising from proximal CHD DS.

percutaneous approach of biliary stenting in patients with PSC. A recent European multicenter randomized 65 patients with PSC with DS to EBD (n = 31) or stent placement for a maximum of 2 weeks (n = 34). Although the cumulative recurrence-free patency of primary DS did not differ significantly between the 2 groups (EBS 0.34 vs 0.30 EBD at 24 months; P = 1.0), much higher adverse events were observed in those who underwent stenting (45% vs 6.7%; odds ratio (OR): 11.7; 95% CI: 2.4–57.2; P = .001).[32] These RCT results further support EBD over short-term EBS as a superior strategy to manage DS, more so in patients with intact papilla.[32] Henceforth, most societal guidelines endorse EBD as the preferred modality but leave the final decision (EBD vs EBS) at the discretion of endoscopist and clinical scenario. Occasionally current endoscopic accessories may fail to pass through a stricture requiring creative and outside-of-the-box approaches by endoscopists. Simons-Linares and colleagues recently managed a severe biliary PSC stricture using a 3-mm percutaneous transluminal coronary angioplasty balloon mounted on a 3-French catheter.[33]

A recent 30-year retrospective analysis of 286 patients from a single German center, with almost 50% distribution of scheduled ERCP and on-demand ERCP suggested a higher transplant-free survival rate (51% vs 29.3%; P<.001) and transplant-free survival time (median: 17.9 vs 15.2 years; log-rank: P = .008) with scheduled ERCP after a mean follow-up of 9.9 years.[34] It is nevertheless noteworthy that because ERCP is a high-risk procedure with a significant adverse event profile, especially in patients with PSC, routine scheduled ERCP is not recommended by major society guidelines.

Role of endoscopic retrograde cholangiopancreatography as a screening tool for cholangiocarcinoma in patients with primary sclerosing cholangitis

Patients with PSC have a 400-fold increased lifetime risk of developing CCA, and this neoplasm accounts for almost one-third of all-cause mortality in these patients.[35] However, there is no consensus regarding a suitable modality to screen patients with PSC for CCA, and performing routine ERCP ± brushing is currently not recommended by any major societal guidelines. The need for ERCP is based on clinical and biochemical deterioration, as well as ductal changes in radiological imaging such as MRCP. If ERCP is undertaken, brushings for cytology + FISH should be sent, and biopsies should be considered for all DS to exclude CCA (see **Fig. 3D–F**). A recent study showed that SOC is effective in establishing an early diagnosis of CCA in PSC based on characteristic morphologic features (see **Fig. 3**), although the morphology of CCA in PSC was quite varied.[28] In addition to neovascularization (see **Fig. 2F**), which is also a hallmark of CCA in the absence of PSC, some cases demonstrated features unique to PSC such as frond-like growths at the hilum (see **Fig. 3E, F**), and others showed intraductal papillary mucinous neoplasms of the bile ducts (IPMN-B) (see **Fig. 3D**), and hence targeted biopsies should be obtained during cholangioscopy. Patients with DS without malignancy were reliably differentiated from CCA in this series of patients with PSC based on cholangioscopic examination.[28]

Endoscopic retrograde cholangiopancreatography-related adverse events in patients with primary sclerosing cholangitis

Therapeutic ERCP in patients with PSC carries a higher complication profile due to the multifocal nature of the disease and intrahepatic bile duct obstruction. A retrospective analysis of ERCPs performed on 168 PSC and 981 patients with non–PSC alluded that while the overall complication rate between the two groups was not significantly different (18/168 (11%) versus 76/981(8%), P = .2), 10% of complications in patients with PSC necessitated hospitalization.[36] Despite antibiotic use before the procedure in patients with PSC, the incidence of cholangitis was higher in the PSC group (4% vs 0.2%, P<.0002).[36] According to the data from a Swedish nationwide quality registry from 51 centers (8932 patients with ERCP; 141 with PSC), patients with PSC had higher overall complications (18.4% vs 7.3%), pancreatitis (7.8% vs 3.2%, $P = .002$), cholangitis (7.1% vs 2.1%, $P < .001$) (see **Fig. 3**C), and perioperative extravasation of contrast (5.7% vs 0.7%, $P < .001$).[37] Furthermore, PSC was estimated to be an independent risk factor for each of these adverse events: pancreatitis (OR: 2.02, 95% CI: 1.04–3.94), cholangitis (OR: 2.88, 95% CI: 1.47–5.65), and extravasation of contrast (OR: 5.84, 95% CI: 2.24–15.23).[37] On the other hand, the Cleveland Clinic retrospective analysis on their 294 patients with PSC who underwent 657 ERCPs from 1998 to 2012, suggested lower overall rates of adverse events (4.3%), with post–ERCP pancreatitis in 8 (1.2%), cholangitis in 16 (2.4%), and bleeding in 4 (0.7%) procedures.[38] Their multivariate analysis identified the performance of sphincterotomy (OR: 5.04, 95% CI: 2.01–12.60; $P = .001$) and passage of the guidewire into the PD (OR: 4.54, 95% CI: 1.44–14.30; $P = .10$) as independent risk factors for adverse events in patients with PSC undergoing ERCP.[38] However, one could argue that sphincterotomy may also have a protective effect for providing easier access for future endoscopic interventions, including passage of larger accessories such as a cholangioscope.[39] Others have reported EBD for stricture, cirrhosis, and low endoscopist volume as predictive risk factors for complications after therapeutic ERCP in patients with PSC.[40]

Endoscopists have adapted various techniques to limit post–ERCP complications in patients with PSC. The use of prophylactic antibiotics is standard practice for ERCP in patients with PSC, and is endorsed by several endoscopic societies.[41] Navaneethan and colleagues have suggested strategies of biliary aspiration immediately after cannulation, aspiration of the contrast postdilation, and avoidance of stenting after the dilation of strictures to be associated with decreased risk of cholangitis (2.1% vs 10.3%; $P = .38$) and major adverse events (2.1% vs 10.3%; $P = .38$).[42] Interestingly, a retrospective analysis of 2000 ERCPs in 931 patients with PSC in Finland between 2009 and 2018 showed that rectal diclofenac was not protective against post–ERCP pancreatitis in patients with PSC, and calls for a future randomized investigation.[43]

IgG-4-related sclerosing cholangitis

IgG-4 cholangiopathy causes concentric bile duct thickening with associated biliary strictures, resulting in chronic cholestasis.[44] Multi-focal central bile duct strictures with associated mild proximal dilation despite a long stricture and bile duct wall thickening with visible lumen are findings suggestive of ISC on ERCP.[3,45] The cornerstone of ISC treatment is corticosteroids (CSs), whereas ERCP is helpful for diagnosis by allowing tissue sampling for histology and immunohistochemical staining, as well as for relieving obstruction with biliary stenting.[45]

Miyazawa and colleagues evaluated 69 patients with ISC (41 managed with CS alone; 28 had additional EBS) and noted that 10/28 (35.7%) patients with EBS experienced spontaneous stent dislodgement after initiating CS.[46] Intentional stent removal was performed in 13 (46.4%) after confirming CS-induced improvement, and 11/13 (84.6%) within 1 month of CS initiation and none of them suffered early (within 2 weeks) recurrence of obstructive jaundice.[46] Of 41 patients managed with CS alone, 10 had obstructive jaundice at the time of CS initiation and all of them achieved clinical improvement without biliary infection.[46] Long-term biliary stenting was noted to be a risk factor for biliary stone/debris development.[46] Based on these data, the authors recommended limiting stent placement to avoid stone formation and considering the removal of biliary stents 2 weeks after the initiation of steroid therapy to prevent stent dislodgement.[46] Similarly, Kuraishi and colleagues enrolled 59 patients with ISC biliary stricture exhibiting jaundice/liver dysfunction who were treated with EBS and noted that the incidence of recurrent biliary obstruction was significantly lower in cases treated with concomitant CS than in those without (1-month no-cholangitis rate 100% vs 90%).[47] These authors also advocated for stent removal within 1 month of initiating CS treatment.[47]

Cholangioscopy in patients with ISC is remarkable for typical features including dilated and tortuous vessels and an absence of partially enlarged vessels.[48] The authors noted a higher incidence of partially enlarged vessels in "distal" CCA than in ISC, increased scarring and pseudo-diverticula in PSC than in ISC, whereas the incidence of dilated/tortuous vessels is significantly higher in ISC than in "hilar" CCA.[45] Although this study defined cholangioscopic features helpful to differentiate ISC from PSC, the authors also suggested monitoring the patterns of proliferative vessels maybe useful in differentiating ISC from CCA.[45]

Choledocholithiasis-associated cholestasis

ERCP is the gold standard for the treatment of CBD stones, but carries an adverse event profile that includes pancreatitis, perforation, and bleeding in 6% to 15% of patients.[49] Data support a high sensitivity ($\sim$89.5%), specificity ($\sim$96.5%), positive predictive value ($\sim$91.9%), and negative predictive value ($\sim$95.3%) of endoscopic ultrasound (EUS) in comparison to ERCP for the diagnosis of CBD stones, emphasizing that ERCP could be avoided in cases of a negative or normal EUS, to limit complications.[50] Procedures taking over 40 min pose increased risks of complications, resulting in unplanned or prolongation of hospitalization (risk ratio (RR): 1.41) and pancreatitis (RR: 1.74).[51] A systematic review (5 RCT, 644 patients) of patients with gallstone pancreatitis showed that early routine ERCP was only effective in reducing mortality and limiting local and systemic complications of pancreatitis in patients with cholangitis (RR: 0.2, 0.45, and 0.37) and/or biliary obstruction (RR: 0.5, 0.53, and 0.56),[52] hence endorsed by societal guidelines. In general, if choledocholithiasis results in cholangitis, early ERCP (within 24 hours) is recommended to facilitate faster recovery, decrease the duration of antibiotic therapy, reduce the duration of hospital stay, and lower morbidity/mortality.[53]

Factors such as older age, previous biliary intervention, elevated serum total bilirubin, large stones, choledocholithiasis above the level of the confluence of the hepatic ducts, stones retained in the cystic duct or Mirizzi syndrome, dilation of the bile duct diagnosed during ERCP, and the need for suprapapillary opening for access are associated with ERCP failure in the achievement of complete CBD clearance and may result in prolonged cholestasis.[54]

According to the American Society of Gastrointestinal Endoscopy (ASGE), for large stones (size $\geq$ 10 mm), endoscopic sphincterotomy followed by large balloon dilation yields higher likelihood of complete bile duct clearance, in comparison to sphincterotomy alone (pooled OR: 2.8; 95% CI: 1.4–5.7).[49] Of 58 studies included in conceptualizing this guideline, the pooled proportion of patients with complete stone extraction was the same in those who underwent lithotripsy or conventional ERCP with balloon sphincteroplasty.[49]

If balloon dilation fails to retrieve the impacted stone and lithotripsy tools or expertise are not available, the next step would be biliary stent placement to restore bile flow to improve cholestasis. Biliary stent placement, rather than initial duct clearance, may be considered for patients who have cholangitis and are hemodynamically unstable in an effort to limit ERCP duration and bacterial translocation during biliary intervention. Traditionally, the biliary stent is left in place for a limited time (few weeks to months) to avoid stent–stone complex formation. Independent risk factors for stent–stone complex formation are long-term ($\geq$301 days) PS placement and increase in CBD diameter.[55] However, contrasting results were reported from a multicenter retrospective study of 83 patients with biliary stents retained for greater than 6 months than 225 in whom stents were removed early, and noted similar overall complications during the 12-month follow-up period (6% vs 4.9%).[56] Biliary stenting can significantly reduce the stone recurrence rate (OR: 0.30; $P = .004$) post–ERCP stone removal and ERCP with assisted lithotripsy.[57] Although, a clear consensus on the safe length of retaining the biliary stent is lacking, most experts advocate for removing the stent within 2 to 3 months.

Secondary sclerosing cholangitis

Progressive cholestatic liver injury in patients without underlying liver disease can lead to SSC, the potential etiologies of which include IsC in critically ill patients, drug-induced cholangiopathy, and autoimmune-mediated mechanisms.[58] SSC in critically ill patients is thought to occur due to a combination of IsC and change in bile composition (toxic bile), which together result in cholangiocyte necrosis and biliary cast formation.[59]

Diagnosis of SSC/IsC is usually established using noninvasive imaging (MRI/MRCP), which displays PSC-like diffuse strictures and dilations of the intrahepatic bile ducts, and often filling defects such as biliary casts.[60] Although ERCP may offer additional advantages such as tissue sampling, bile aspiration for microbiological evaluation, and bile flow restoration with therapeutic interventions such as balloon dilation or endoluminal stenting, most studies report a delay in performing ERCP in IsC up to 60 days.[61] This delay is due to several interplaying factors, including the patient being unstable/critically-ill for ERCP, mis-diagnosis with cholestasis of sepsis, and presence of bile duct dilation in less than 50% of critically ill patients with IsC.[61]

When performed, ERCP cholangiography in IsC may show filling defects in intrahepatic bile ducts (biliary casts), progressive destruction/obliteration of intrahepatic bile ducts, and a central biliary system with "pruned tree" appearance.[62] Although IsC mainly occurs in the intrahepatic bile ducts, involvement of extrahepatic ducts (6%), as well as concomitant involvement of both intrahepatic and extrahepatic bile ducts (20%) has been reported.[62] During ERCP in patients with IsC, adequate sampling for microbiological evaluation is advised as a pathogen has been reported to grow in almost 98% of cases and pathogen identification may help guide antibiotic therapy.[63]

Infection-related cholangiopathy

AIDS-cholangiopathy is an uncommon cause of SSC, seen in patients with advanced human immunodeficiency virus (HIV) and CD4 counts less than $10/mm^3$, the incidence of which has significantly declined over the past few decades, mainly due to advances in antiretroviral therapy (ART). AIDS-cholangiopathy typically presents with stricture of distal CBD and papillary stenosis.[3] However, diffuse irregularity in the caliber of the intrahepatic bile ducts may be seen in a subset of patients.[64] Additionally, concomitant infection by cytomegalovirus (CMV), microsporidium, or cryptosporidium has been reported in cases with intrahepatic duct involvement.[64]

For AIDS-cholangiopathy, the mainstay of management is the control of ongoing opportunistic infection with appropriate antiviral or antibiotic therapy, as well as the restoration of the immune system with ART. Patients with symptomatic cholangitis, with abdominal pain and jaundice, show almost immediate relief with sphincterotomy.[64,65] However, sphincterotomy has not been shown to be effective in the normalization of alkaline phosphatase (ALP) long-term or preventing progression to intrahepatic sclerosing cholangitis.[65] Isolated strictures could be treated with temporary EBS.

Recurrent pyogenic cholangitis (RPC) is predominantly seen in Southeast Asia, wherein as the result of recurrent biliary infections (usually bacterial), intrahepatic, and extrahepatic biliary strictures with scarring occurs, resulting in intraductal pigment stone formation.[66] Dilated intrahepatic and extrahepatic bile ducts with minimally dilated peripheral bile ducts, and associated multiple ductal stones should favor a diagnosis of RPC during ERCP, as opposed to PSC.[66] ERCP is the preferred therapeutic approach for RPC that is predominantly localized to the extrahepatic biliary system, especially CBD/CHD for stone clearance with a high success rate (~91.7%).[67] Although, hepatectomy is ultimately indicated in most RPC cases, ERCP has an important role for relief in biliary obstruction and cholestasis. Other less common infections resulting in biliary cholestasis may include helminths (viz. Ascariasis, Fascioliasis, Schistosomiasis, Clonorchis, Strongyloidiasis, Capillariasis, Opisthorchiasis, Visceral larva migrans) and protozoans (viz. Leishmaniasis, Toxoplasmosis), but are less common in the western world, although occasionally encountered especially in immigrant populations (**Fig. 4**). These infections can cause biliary obstruction, cholangitis, and additionally chronic cholestasis.[68]

Post–liver transplant biliary stricture-related cholestasis

One of the commonest complications postorthotopic liver transplant (OLT) is anastomotic biliary stricture (ABS), resulting in cholestasis. ABS is more common with live donor liver transplant, as opposed to deceased donor LT (10%–37% vs 5%–15%, respectively).[69] The preferred approach for the management of post–OLT ABS includes ERCP with EBD followed by the placement of PSs or fully covered self-expandable metallic stent (FC-SEMS).[69] Monotherapy with EBD has higher chance of recurrence over time than dilation/stenting approach (62% vs 31%).[70]

PSs have higher associated complication profile, including stent occlusion and requirement of frequent endoscopic sessions. The overall success rate of post–OLT ABS management with EBD and PS placement is 80% to 95%,[71] and similar overall

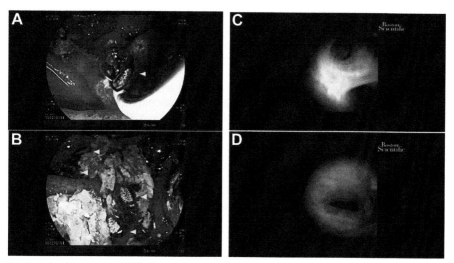

Fig. 4. Infectious cause of cholestatic liver disease (Liver fluke) – (*A*): ERCP removal of liver fluke from CBD; (*B*): multiple liver flukes and associated debris/pus; (*C*): cholangioscopy with impacted liver fluke in R main hepatic duct; (*D*): cholangioscopy with edematous appearance of CBD after fluke clearance.

success has been reported with FC-SEMS (85%–95%) as well.[72] Sung and colleagues reported higher functional (100% vs 80%, P = .005) and radiological (100% vs 70%, P = .07) resolution of biliary obstruction with FC-SEMS than patients who received PS; however, there was no difference in 1-year recurrence rate.[69] Many of the limitations associated with PS may be overcome by the use of multiple plastic stents (MPSs), to achieve greater dilation effect, and less stent occlusion. A recent metanalysis of 4 RCTs with 205 patients with post–OLT ABS showed that resolution (OR: 1.05, 95% CI: 0.43–2.56, P = .92), recurrence (OR: 2.37, 95%CI: 0.54–10.38, P = .25), adverse events (OR: 0.91, 95%CI: 0.84–3.48, P = .86), and stent migration rate (OR: 1.31, 95%CI: 0.46–3.71, P = .61) were not statistically different between patients with MPS versus FC-SEMS approach,[73] although FC-SEMS group had fewer ERCPs performed (mean difference = 2.08).[73]

Optimal time interval between stent exchanges has been investigated in multiple studies. Morelli and colleagues prospectively evaluated 38 patients with post–OLT ABS with ERCP-EBD and stent placement every 2 weeks.[74] The authors reported the mean number of ERCPs per patient 3.4 (range 2–6), mean number of maximum stents placed 2.5 (range 1–6) and mean total stenting period 107 days (range 20–198 days), and after a mean follow-up period of 360 days (range 140–1347 days), the long-term stricture resolution was achieved in 33/38 (87%) patients.[74] The authors advocated a rapid sequence endoscopic approach with accelerated dilation and shorter total length of stenting to achieve long-term success in patients with post–OLT ABS.[74] Tabibian and colleagues studied 83 patients with post–OLT ABS, of which 69 completed endoscopic treatment, and then compared 65/69 (94%) with successful resolution and the failures who needed hepaticojejunostomy (HJ).[73] Comparing the resolution group and HJ group, there were, respectively, 8.0 and 3.5 total stents (P = .021), 2.5 and 1.3 stents per ERCP (P = .018) (maximum = 9), 4.2 and 2.8 ERCPs (P = .15), and 20 and 22 months from OLT to ABS diagnosis (P = .19). The authors inferred that treatment success directly correlated with the number of stents used in total and during each ERCP to achieve maximal effective stenting.[75] Most experts advocate for stent exchange within 3 months to avoid long-term stent complications, such as stone/sludge formation within/upstream of the stent or stent migration/blockage resulting in cholangitis.

Recently, Barakat and Girotra and colleagues from Stanford evaluated 77 patients with post–OLT ABS who underwent 277 incremental dilations of stricture and stent exchange (IDSE) and 132 sequential stent addition (SSA) procedures.[76] In IDSE strategy, the previous biliary stents are removed, stricture reassessed and dilated and new multiple stents are placed, whereas in SSA protocol, the previous biliary stents are not removed, and rather the stricture area is dilated and additional stent is added across the NAS. The authors noted 64.5% shorter fluoroscopy time (P<.0001), 41.5% shorter mean procedure duration (P < .0001) with SSA protocol, as well as the use of fewer accessories, resulting in 63.8% lower material and 42.8% lower facility costs, than IDSE. It was noteworthy that the stricture resolution was greater than 95% and low adverse events rates did not significantly differ between the groups.[76] Based on that, the group advocated SSA protocol with shorter, cost-effective procedure, with less radiation exposure to the patient. This is an interesting evolutionary step in the management of post–OLT ABS and needs to be investigated in multicenter randomized approach.

SUMMARY

Intrahepatic and extrahepatic bile duct injuries can result in bile duct obstruction and chronic cholestasis, which if unresolved may progress to the fibrosis and development of cirrhosis. It is important for endoscopists not only to recognize the fluoroscopic, cholangiographic (MRCP/ERCP), and cholangioscopic features indicative of PSC, along with utility and limitations of brush cytology, FISH analysis, and biopsies but also to remain cognizant of subtle vascular/mucosal changes in DSs, which may hint toward early progression to CCA. ERCP also plays a major role in the management of choledocholithiasis, as well as ischemic, autoimmune (IGG4), and infectious cholangiopathies. We are optimistic that increased the utilization of cholangioscopy, when integrated with molecular advances will result in rapid advancements in this field, will allow better definitions of PSC strictures, early and accurate diagnosis of CCA, and overall robust endoscopic management protocols for PSC and other CLDs.

DISCLOSURE

The authors have nothing to disclose.

REFERENCES

1. Gossard AA, Talwalkar JA. Cholestatic liver disease. Med Clin North Am 2014;98: 73–85.
2. Vlăduț C, Ciocîrlan M, Bilous D, et al. An overview on primary sclerosing cholangitis. J Clin Med 2020;9:754.
3. Role of endoscopy in primary sclerosing cholangitis: European society of Gastrointestinal endoscopy (ESGE) and European association for the study of the liver (EASL) clinical guideline. J Hepatol 2017;66:1265–81.
4. Weber C, Kuhlencordt R, Grotelueschen R, et al. Magnetic resonance cholangiopancreatography in the diagnosis of primary sclerosing cholangitis. Endoscopy 2008;40:739–45.
5. Hammel P, Couvelard A, O'Toole D, et al. Regression of liver fibrosis after biliary drainage in patients with chronic pancreatitis and stenosis of the common bile duct. N Engl J Med 2001;344:418–23.
6. Stiehl A, Rudolph G, Klöters-Plachky P, et al. Development of dominant bile duct stenoses in patients with primary sclerosing cholangitis treated with ursodeoxycholic acid: outcome after endoscopic treatment. J Hepatol 2002;36:151–6.
7. Chapman MH, Webster GJ, Bannoo S, et al. Cholangiocarcinoma and dominant strictures in patients with primary sclerosing cholangitis: a 25-year single-centre experience. Eur J Gastroenterol Hepatol 2012;24:1051–8.
8. Trikudanathan G, Navaneethan U, Njei B, et al. Diagnostic yield of bile duct brushings for cholangiocarcinoma in primary sclerosing cholangitis: a systematic review and meta-analysis. Gastrointest Endosc 2014;79:783–9.
9. Charatcharoenwitthaya P, Enders FB, Halling KC, et al. Utility of serum tumor markers, imaging, and biliary cytology for detecting cholangiocarcinoma in primary sclerosing cholangitis. Hepatology 2008;48:1106–17.
10. Boberg KM, Jebsen P, Clausen OP, et al. Diagnostic benefit of biliary brush cytology in cholangiocarcinoma in primary sclerosing cholangitis. J Hepatol 2006;45:568–74.
11. Witt BL, Kristen Hilden RN, Scaife C, et al. Identification of factors predictive of malignancy in patients with atypical biliary brushing results obtained via ERCP. Diagn Cytopathol 2013;41:682–8.
12. Barr Fritcher EG, Kipp BR, Voss JS, et al. Primary sclerosing cholangitis patients with serial polysomy fluorescence in situ hybridization results are at increased risk of cholangiocarcinoma. Am J Gastroenterol 2011;106:2023–8.

13. Bangarulingam SY, Bjornsson E, Enders F, et al. Long-term outcomes of positive fluorescence in situ hybridization tests in primary sclerosing cholangitis. Hepatology 2010;51:174–80.

14. Navaneethan U, Njei B, Venkatesh PGK, et al. Fluorescence in situ hybridization for diagnosis of cholangiocarcinoma in primary sclerosing cholangitis: a systematic review and meta-analysis. Gastrointest Endosc 2014;79:943–50.e3.

15. Singhi AD, Nikiforova MN, Chennat J, et al. Integrating next-generation sequencing to endoscopic retrograde cholangiopancreatography (ERCP)-obtained biliary specimens improves the detection and management of patients with malignant bile duct strictures. Gut 2020;69:52–61.

16. Franzini TA, Moura RN, de Moura EG. Advances in therapeutic cholangioscopy. Gastroenterol Res Pract 2016;2016:5249152.

17. Njei B, McCarty TR, Varadarajulu S, et al. Systematic review with meta-analysis: endoscopic retrograde cholangiopancreatography-based modalities for the diagnosis of cholangiocarcinoma in primary sclerosing cholangitis. Aliment Pharmacol Ther 2016;44:1139–51.

18. Arnelo U, von Seth E, Bergquist A. Prospective evaluation of the clinical utility of single-operator peroral cholangioscopy in patients with primary sclerosing cholangitis. Endoscopy 2015;47:696–702.

19. Azeem N, Gostout CJ, Knipschield M, et al. Cholangioscopy with narrow-band imaging in patients with primary sclerosing cholangitis undergoing ERCP. Gastrointest Endosc 2014;79:773–9.e2.

20. Ishida Y, Itoi T, Okabe Y. Types of peroral cholangioscopy: how to choose the most suitable type of cholangioscopy. Curr Treat Options Gastroenterol 2016; 14:210–9.

21. Majeed A, Castedal M, Arnelo U, et al. Optimizing the detection of biliary dysplasia in primary sclerosing cholangitis before liver transplantation. Scand J Gastroenterol 2018;53:56–63.

22. Prat F, Leblanc S, Foissac F, et al. Impact of peroral cholangioscopy on the management of indeterminate biliary conditions: a multicentre prospective trial. Frontline Gastroenterol 2019;10:236–43.

23. Han S, Kahaleh M, Sharaiah RZ, et al. Probe-based confocal laser endomicroscopy in the evaluation of dominant strictures in patients with primary sclerosing cholangitis: results of a U.S. multicenter prospective trial. Gastrointest Endosc 2021;94(3):569–76.e1.

24. Lindor KD, Kowdley KV, Harrison EM. ACG clinical guideline: primary sclerosing cholangitis. Am J Gastroenterol 2015;110:646–59.

25. Cazzagon N, Chazouillères O, Corpechot C, et al. Predictive criteria of response to endoscopic treatment for severe strictures in primary sclerosing cholangitis. Clin Res Hepatol Gastroenterol 2019;43:387–94.

26. Chapman MH, Thorburn D, Hirschfield GM, et al. British Society of Gastroenterology and UK-PSC guidelines for the diagnosis and management of primary sclerosing cholangitis. Gut 2019;68:1356–78.

27. Gotthardt DN, Rudolph G, Klöters-Plachky P, et al. Endoscopic dilation of dominant stenoses in primary sclerosing cholangitis: outcome after long-term treatment. Gastrointest Endosc 2010;71:527–34.

28. Tejaswi SLT, Olson KA. Cholangioscopy in primary sclerosing cholangitis: a case series of benign findings. Video GIE 2021;6(6):277–81.

29. van Boeckel PG, Vleggaar FP, Siersema PD. Plastic or metal stents for benign extrahepatic biliary strictures: a systematic review. BMC Gastroenterol 2009;9:96.

30. van Milligen de Wit AW, Rauws EA, van Bracht J, et al. Lack of complications following short-term stent therapy for extrahepatic bile duct strictures in primary sclerosing cholangitis. Gastrointest Endosc 1997;46:344–7.

31. Kaya M, Petersen BT, Angulo P, et al. Balloon dilation compared to stenting of dominant strictures in primary sclerosing cholangitis. Am J Gastroenterol 2001; 96:1059–66.

32. Ponsioen CY, Arnelo U, Bergquist A, et al. No superiority of stents vs balloon dilatation for dominant strictures in patients with primary sclerosing cholangitis. Gastroenterology 2018;155:752–9.e5.

33. Simons-Linares CR, O'Shea R, Chahal P. Severe primary sclerosing cholangitis biliary stricture managed with a small-caliber cardiac angioplasty balloon: looking outside the endoscopic retrograde cholangiopancreatography toolbox. ACG Case Rep J 2019;6:e00141.

34. Rupp C, Hippchen T, Bruckner T, et al. Effect of scheduled endoscopic dilatation of dominant strictures on outcome in patients with primary sclerosing cholangitis. Gut 2019;68:2170–8.

35. Boonstra K, Weersma RK, van Erpecum KJ, et al. Population-based epidemiology, malignancy risk, and outcome of primary sclerosing cholangitis. Hepatology 2013;58:2045–55.

36. Bangarulingam SY, Gossard AA, Petersen BT, et al. Complications of endoscopic retrograde cholangiopancreatography in primary sclerosing cholangitis. Am J Gastroenterol 2009;104:855–60.

37. von Seth E, Arnelo U, Enochsson L, et al. Primary sclerosing cholangitis increases the risk for pancreatitis after endoscopic retrograde cholangiopancreatography. Liver Int 2015;35:254–62.

38. Navaneethan U, Jegadeesan R, Nayak S, et al. ERCP-related adverse events in patients with primary sclerosing cholangitis. Gastrointest Endosc 2015;81:410–9.

39. Ismail S, Kylänpää L, Mustonen H, et al. Risk factors for complications of ERCP in primary sclerosing cholangitis. Endoscopy 2012;44:1133–8.

40. Ahmad J. Metal, magnet or transplant: options in primary sclerosing cholangitis with stricture. Hepatol Int 2018;12:510–9.

41. Khashab MA, Chithadi KV, Acosta RD, et al. Antibiotic prophylaxis for GI endoscopy. Gastrointest Endosc 2015;81:81–9.

42. Navaneethan U, Lourdusamy D, Gutierrez NG, et al. New approach to decrease post-ERCP adverse events in patients with primary sclerosing cholangitis. Endosc Int Open 2017;5:E710–7.

43. Koskensalo V, Tenca A, Udd M, et al. Diclofenac does not reduce the risk of acute pancreatitis in patients with primary sclerosing cholangitis after endoscopic retrograde cholangiography. United Eur Gastroenterol J 2020;8:462–71.

44. Moon SH, Kim MH, Lee JK, et al. Development of a scoring system for differentiating IgG4-related sclerosing cholangitis from primary sclerosing cholangitis. J Gastroenterol 2017;52:483–93.

45. Jung YJ, Moon SH, Kim MH. Role of endoscopic procedures in the diagnosis of IgG4-related pancreatobiliary disease. Chonnam Med J 2021;57:44–50.

46. Miyazawa M, Takatori H, Kawaguchi K, et al. Management of biliary stricture in patients with IgG4-related sclerosing cholangitis. PLoS One 2020;15:e0232089.

47. Kuraishi Y, Muraki T, Ashihara N, et al. Validity and safety of endoscopic biliary stenting for biliary stricture associated with IgG4-related pancreatobiliary disease during steroid therapy. Endosc Int open 2019;7:E1410–8.

48. Itoi T, Kamisawa T, Igarashi Y, et al. The role of peroral video cholangioscopy in patients with IgG4-related sclerosing cholangitis. J Gastroenterol 2013;48: 504–14.
49. Buxbaum JL, Abbas Fehmi SM, Sultan S, et al. ASGE guideline on the role of endoscopy in the evaluation and management of choledocholithiasis. Gastrointest Endosc 2019;89:1075–105.e15.
50. Anwer M, Asghar MS, Rahman S, et al. Diagnostic accuracy of endoscopic ultrasonography versus the gold standard endoscopic retrograde cholangiopancreatography in detecting common bile duct stones. Cureus 2020;12:e12162.
51. Turbayne AKB, Mehta A, Thomson A. Prolonged endoscopic retrograde cholangiopancreatography results in higher rates of pancreatitis and unplanned hospitalisation. Surg Endosc 2021. https://doi.org/10.1007/s00464-021-08488-w.
52. Tse F, Yuan Y. Early routine endoscopic retrograde cholangiopancreatography strategy versus early conservative management strategy in acute gallstone pancreatitis. Cochrane Database Syst Rev 2012;(5):Cd009779.
53. Florescu V, Pârvuleţu R, Ardelean M, et al. The emergency endoscopic treatment in acute cholangitis. Chirurgia (Bucur) 2021;116:42–50.
54. Marcelino LP, Thofehrn S, Eyff TF, et al. Factors predictive of the successful treatment of choledocholithiasis. Surg Endosc 2021. https://doi.org/10.1007/s00464-021-08463-5.
55. Kaneko J, Kawata K, Watanabe S, et al. Clinical characteristics and risk factors for stent-stone complex formation following biliary plastic stent placement in patients with common bile duct stones. J Hepatobiliary Pancreat Sci 2018;25: 448–54.
56. Sbeit W, Khoury T, Kadah A, et al. Long-term safety of endoscopic biliary stents for cholangitis complicating choledocholithiasis: a multi-center study. J Clin Med 2020;9:2953.
57. Choi JH, Lee TY, Cheon YK. Effect of stent placement on stone recurrence and post-procedural cholangitis after endoscopic removal of common bile duct stones. Korean J Intern Med 2021;36:S27–34.
58. Edwards K, Allison M, Ghuman S. Secondary sclerosing cholangitis in critically ill patients: a rare disease precipitated by severe SARS-CoV-2 infection. BMJ Case Rep 2020;13:e237984.
59. Leonhardt S, Veltzke-Schlieker W, Adler A, et al. Trigger mechanisms of secondary sclerosing cholangitis in critically ill patients. Crit Care 2015;19:131.
60. Laurent L, Lemaitre C, Minello A, et al. Cholangiopathy in critically ill patients surviving beyond the intensive care period: a multicentre survey in liver units. Aliment Pharmacol Ther 2017;46:1070–6.
61. Martins P, Verdelho Machado M. Secondary sclerosing cholangitis in critically ill patients: an underdiagnosed Entity. GE Port J Gastroenterol 2020;27:103–14.
62. Leonhardt S, Veltzke-Schlieker W, Adler A, et al. Secondary sclerosing cholangitis in critically ill patients: clinical Presentation, cholangiographic features, natural history, and outcome: a series of 16 cases. Medicine (Baltimore) 2015;94:e2188.
63. Kirchner GI, Rümmele P. Update on sclerosing cholangitis in critically ill patients. Viszeralmedizin 2015;31:178–84.
64. Benhamou Y, Caumes E, Gerosa Y, et al. AIDS-related cholangiopathy. Critical analysis of a prospective series of 26 patients. Dig Dis Sci 1993;38:1113–8.
65. Cello JP, Chan MF. Long-term follow-up of endoscopic retrograde cholangiopancreatography sphincterotomy for patients with acquired immune deficiency syndrome papillary stenosis. Am J Med 1995;99:600–3.

66. Kwan KEL, Shelat VG, Tan CH. Recurrent pyogenic cholangitis: a review of imaging findings and clinical management. Abdom Radiol (NY) 2017;42:46–56.
67. Lam SK. A study of endoscopic sphincterotomy in recurrent pyogenic cholangitis. Br J Surg 1984;71:262–6.
68. Case records of the Massachusetts General Hospital. Weekly clinicopathological exercises. Case 28-2001. A 44-year-old woman with chills, fever, jaundice, and hepatic abscesses. N Engl J Med 2001;345:817–23.
69. Sung MJ, Jo JH, Lee HS, et al. Optimal drainage of anastomosis stricture after living donor liver transplantation. Surg Endosc 2021. https://doi.org/10.1007/s00464-021-08456-4.
70. Zoepf T, Maldonado-Lopez EJ, Hilgard P, et al. Balloon dilatation vs. balloon dilatation plus bile duct endoprostheses for treatment of anastomotic biliary strictures after liver transplantation. Liver Transpl 2006;12:88–94.
71. Boeva I, Karagyozov PI, Tishkov I. Post-liver transplant biliary complications: current knowledge and therapeutic advances. World J Hepatol 2021;13:66–79.
72. Villa NA, Harrison ME. Management of biliary strictures after liver transplantation. Gastroenterol Hepatol (N Y) 2015;11:316–28.
73. Tringali A, Tarantino I, Barresi L, et al. Multiple plastic versus fully covered metal stents for managing post-liver transplantation anastomotic biliary strictures: a meta-analysis of randomized controlled trials. Ann Gastroenterol 2019;32:407–15.
74. Morelli G, Fazel A, Judah J, et al. Rapid-sequence endoscopic management of posttransplant anastomotic biliary strictures. Gastrointest Endosc 2008;67:879–85.
75. Tabibian JH, Asham EH, Han S, et al. Endoscopic treatment of postorthotopic liver transplantation anastomotic biliary strictures with maximal stent therapy (with video). Gastrointest Endosc 2010;71:505–12.
76. Barakat MT, Huang RJ, Thosani NC, et al. Liver transplant-related anastomotic biliary strictures: a novel, rapid, safe, radiation-sparing, and cost-effective management approach. Gastrointest Endosc 2018;87:501–8.

Improving Diagnostic Yield in Indeterminate Biliary Strictures

David J. Restrepo, MD[a], Chris Moreau, BSBME[b],
Cyrus V. Edelson, MD[c], Ameesh Dev, MD[d],
Shreyas Saligram, MD, MRCP (UK)[b], Hari Sayana, MD[b],
Sandeep N. Patel, DO[b,*]

KEYWORDS

- (Mesh): bile ducts • Cholestasis • Constriction • Pathologic
- Cholangiopancreatography • Endoscopic retrograde
- Biliary tract surgical procedures

KEY POINTS

- Indeterminate biliary strictures pose a diagnostic challenge when trying to determine if a biliary stricture is of malignant or benign origin.
- Indeterminate biliary strictures can lead to a delay in urgent surgical resection or to unnecessary morbid surgeries.
- Emerging technologies which include imaging, laboratory tests, and tissue sampling techniques aid in the differentiation of these complex cases.

INTRODUCTION

A bile duct stricture is defined as a narrowing of the bile duct, by either extrinsic compression or pathophysiological internal lumen reduction, reducing the ability for bile to flow from the liver to the duodenum. It can be caused by different clinical conditions that can be benign or malignant in nature. Benign strictures are more common

Financial Disclosure Statement: This study was not funded by any institution or individual.
[a] Department of Medicine, Division of Internal Medicine, University of Texas Health San Antonio, 7703 Floyd Curl Drive, San Antonio, TX 78229, USA; [b] Department of Medicine, Division of Gastroenterology, University of Texas Health San Antonio, 7703 Floyd Curl Drive, San Antonio, TX 78229, USA; [c] Department of Medicine, Division of Gastroenterology, Brooke Army Medical Center, 3551 Roger Brooke Drive, Fort Sam, Houston, TX 78234, USA; [d] School of Medicine, University of Texas Health San Antonio, 7703 Floyd Curl Drive, San Antonio, TX 78229, USA
* Corresponding author. University of Texas Health Science Center at San Antonio, 7703 Floyd Curl Drive, MC 7858, San Antonio, TX 78229.
E-mail address: Patels7@uthscsa.edu

Clin Liver Dis 26 (2022) 69–80
https://doi.org/10.1016/j.cld.2021.08.007
1089-3261/22/© 2021 Elsevier Inc. All rights reserved.

than malignant strictures, and their causes frequently include chronic pancreatitis, iatrogenic injuries, ston-induced strictures, autoimmune diseases, primary sclerosing cholangitis, as well as other pathologies. The more common causes of malignant strictures include pancreatic ductal adenocarcinoma and cholangiocarcinoma, whereas less common causes are ampullary malignancies, gallbladder tumors, and metastatic cancer.[1] The etiology of malignant bile duct strictures can vary depending on the anatomic site at which the obstruction occurs. For instance, the proximal and mid bile ducts are more commonly obstructed by intrahepatic and extrahepatic cholangiocarcinomas. However, distal malignant bile duct obstructions are more frequently caused by pancreatic ductal adenocarcinoma. Unfortunately, only 30% of malignant biliary strictures are resectable when identified.[2] The most challenging biliary strictures to diagnose are those which cannot easily be definitively defined as malignant or benign, known as indeterminate biliary strictures.

Indeterminate biliary strictures are defined as strictures associated with negative diagnostic workups, usually including cross-sectional imaging and endoscopic retrograde cholangiopancreatography (ERCP) with standard multimodal tissue sampling. Confirming stricture etiology is required for appropriate, personalized treatments, and avoidance of delay in care.[3] Data have shown that up to two-thirds of indeterminate biliary strictures are of malignant origin and 15% to 24% of all surgical resections for a presumptively malignant indeterminate biliary obstruction have a benign pathology.[2]

Improving diagnostic yield in indeterminate biliary strictures is essential to avoid delays in resection and morbidity due to unnecessary surgical procedures. We will review and discuss recent literature on techniques and tools that aid the diagnosis of indeterminate biliary obstructions.

Physical examination and history

Bile duct strictures have a wide spectrum of clinical presentations ranging from completely asymptomatic to jaundice, pruritus, and ascending cholangitis. Thorough history and chronology of presentation can provide diagnostic clues suggestive of malignant strictures. Special attention should be given to symptoms indicative of malignant strictures, such as fevers, chills, night sweats, unintentional weight loss, decrease in appetite, back pain, unexplained abdominal pain, and fatigue. One should also assess for cachexia and palpable abdominal masses on physical examination. Evaluation of liver function using established serum biomarkers should be performed in conjunction with the physical examination.

Laboratory workup

Bilirubin, alkaline phosphatase, and liver enzymes

Regardless of etiology, patients with biliary strictures often have abnormal liver-associated enzymes in a cholestatic pattern. If unclear, this should be confirmed with additional testing such as alkaline phosphatase isoenzymes or gamma-glutamyl transferase. Furthermore, elevated bilirubin is a greater predictor of malignant strictures than other liver-associated enzymes.[4–8] When malignancy is suspected, tumor biomarkers may be considered during evaluation.

Tumor markers

Serum cancer antigen 19 to 9 (CA19-9) and carcinoembryonic antigen (CEA) are frequently measured in patients with a suspected biliary stricture. CA19 to 9 remains a controversial test in differentiating between malignant and benign biliary strictures. It has been shown to be elevated in patients with benign conditions, specifically those with benign biliary strictures. However, serum CA19 to 9 results will rarely be the deciding factor when considering surgical intervention in patients with indeterminate biliary strictures.[9] Conditions other than biliary malignant obstructions such as cirrhosis, stomach cancer, cholangitis, and cholestasis can also elevate CA 19 to 9 levels.

CEA is rarely used as a diagnostic tool due to its low performance in patients with indeterminate biliary strictures.[10] Other markers such as transthyretin, matrix metalloproteinase 7, and microRNA-16 have been studied, but their use in patients with indeterminate biliary strictures is limited and not currently recommended. Initial testing for tumor markers can aid in narrowing the differential of stricture etiology; however, testing rarely confirms the diagnosis due to the limited sensitivity and specificity of these tumor markers.[10]

Radiological evaluation

Due to its noninvasive nature, radiologic evaluation is typically the first step in working up a biliary stricture. Transabdominal ultrasound, computed tomography (CT), magnetic resonance imaging (MRI) of the abdomen, and magnetic resonance cholangiopancreatography (MRCP) are typically used for the evaluation of patients with suspected biliary strictures. Information on the role of imaging in diagnosing indeterminate biliary strictures is scarce. This is likely because these tests do not allow for tissue diagnosis, but rather the detection of an obstruction. Although certain radiologic characteristics can favor benign or malignant etiology, its specificity can be aberrant as seen in **Table 1**.

ENDOSCOPIC WORKUP
Endoscopic ultrasound

Endoscopic ultrasound (EUS) is one of the cornerstone examinations available for the evaluation of indeterminate biliary strictures. It is a particularly useful tool when cross-sectional imaging shows a stricture that is caused by extrinsic compression and there is no clinical indication for biliary decompression.[11] The EUS probe can be maneuvered into the stomach or duodenum to evaluate the bile duct with real-time imaging, and both radial and linear views are available depending on the probe selected. Additionally, linear probes allow for tissue sampling through fine-needle aspiration (FNA) of tumors and surrounding lymph nodes which can provide a diagnosis as well as staging in the case of malignancy.[12,13] Due to the risk of seeding, we do not perform EUS–FNA in our practice for patients that are considered potential surgical candidates but it has been described in the literature. EUS–FNA may offer a better evaluation of extrahepatic bile duct pathology than the hilum and more proximal bile ducts. A 2011 single-center retrospective trial showed a sensitivity of 73% for the diagnosis of cholangiocarcinoma by EUS–FNA. Of note, when comparing the distal and proximal ducts, there was a statistically significant difference in sensitivities with distal being 81% versus 59% in the proximal.[14] Furthermore, EUS–FNA for distal strictures has been reported to increase sensitivity from 33% to 93% in cytology negative strictures.[15] This result is in line with a meta-analysis published in 2019 which concluded that EUS increases the identification of malignancy for indeterminate biliary strictures following a nondiagnostic ERCP, particularly those that are distal or related to extrinsic compression.[16]

Endoscopic retrograde cholangiopancreatography

ERCP is the most commonly used modality to identify, sample, and treat intrahepatic and extrahepatic biliary strictures.[17,18] It is indicated when cross-sectional imaging shows a thickened bile duct, neoplastic lesions with intraductal invasion, or when

Table 1
Overview of sensitivity and specificity in the malignancy detection of different diagnostic modalities for indeterminate biliary strictures

Modality			
Radiological Evaluation	**Obstruction Detection Sensitivity (%)**	**Benign vs Malignant Classification Specificity (%)**	**Reference**
US	90–95	30–70	56
CT	>90	60–90	2,56
MRI	95–98	30–90	2,57–59
EUS + FNA (proximal)	76% (95% CI: 66%–85%)	100% (95% CI: 95%–100%)	60
EUS + FNA (distal)	83% (95% CI: 68%–98%)	100% (95% CI: 63%–100%)	60
Endocospic Studies	**Sensitivity for Malignancy Detection (%)**	**Specificity for Malignancy Detection (%)**	**Reference**
ERCP + Brushing Cytology	45 (95% CI: 40–50)	99 (95% CI 98–100)	20
ERCP + Intraductal Biopsy	48 (95% CI: 42–53)	99 (95% CI 98–100)	20
ERCP + Brushing Cytology + Intraductal Biopsy	59 (95% CI: 53.7–64.8)	100 (95% CI 99–100)	20
Cholangioscopy Visual Diagnosis	94 (95% CI: 89–97) / 87	95 (95% CI: 90–98) / 71.2	32 / 33
Cholangioscopy + Spyglass Biopsy	88 / 75	94 / 100	61 / 33
Cholangioscopy + Biopsy + Aspiration Fluid Cytology	81[a]–94[b]	79[b]–100[a]	62
pCLE	89 (95% CI: 79–95) / 98	71% (95% CI: 54–84) / 67	44 / 63
OCT	Not enough data	Not enough data	
IDUS	0.93 (95% CI: 0.90–0.97)	0.89 (95% CI: 0.85–0.94)	48
Molecular			
FISH	44 / 39 / 41	99 / 100 / 100	15 / 53 / 54
FISH + Cytology	54 / 51 / 61	98 / 100 / 100	15 / 53 / 54
MP	50 / 39	97 / 100	53 / 54
MP + Cytology	63 / 59	97 / 100	53 / 54
FISH + MP	55 / 61	99 / 97	15 / 53
FISH + MP + Cytology	63 / 69 / 78	98 / 97 / 100	15 / 53 / 54

Abbreviations: CI, confidence interval; CT, computed tomography; ERCP, endoscopic retrograde cholangiopancreatography; EUS, endoscopic ultrasound; FISH, fluorescent in situ hybridization; FNA, fine-needle aspiration; IDUS, intraductal ultrasound; MP, mutation profiling; MRI, magnetic resonance imaging; OCT, optical coherence tomography; pCLE, probe-based confocal laser endomicroscopy.

[a] Atypical cells as benign.
[b] Atypical cells as malignant.

biliary decompression is clinically indicated.[11] ERCP allows for several techniques for obtaining tissue samples; brushing, intraductal forceps biopsy, biliary aspirate, and stent removal with cytopathological analysis.[19] In 2015, Navaneethan and colleagues published a meta-analysis reviewing pooled sensitivity and specificity for brushing and forceps biopsy. For brushing, it reported a pooled sensitivity of 45% and 99% sensitivity, whereas intraductal biopsy reported 48% sensitivity and 99% specificity. When both techniques were combined, sensitivity increased to 59% and specificity remained at 100%.[20] Various strategies have been found to increase the yield of this diagnostic modality, such as longer brushes,[21] increased number of passes, dilating the stenosis before brushing,[22] and fluorescent in situ hybridization (FISH).[15] Additionally, studies have shown that combining brush cytology with bile aspiration and/or fluoroscopically directed forceps biopsy can improve sensitivity.[19]

Bile aspiration may also increase diagnostic yield when combined with ERCP brushing. One study tested bile duct aspirate in conjunction with brush cytology, and it reported an increase in sensitivity from 20% to 54%.[23] Moreover, strategies like collecting the bile duct aspirate after disrupting the bile duct mucosa have also been shown to further increase sensitivity. In one study, it was shown that postbrushing lavage fluid yielded a sensitivity of 70% for malignant bile duct strictures.[24]

Single-operator cholangioscopy

Single-operator cholangioscopy (SOC) is a relatively new technology that works by directly visualizing the bile duct.[25] This allows for the direct visual evaluation of the bile duct and ease of targeting for biopsy collection at the site of the stricture. There are different types of cholangioscopes, including dual operator, single operator, and direct per oral cholangioscopy. The first cholangioscopes were fiber optic devices that offered direct intraductal visualization. Those have been replaced with a digital single-operator system (SpyGlass, Boston Scientific Corp, Massachusetts, USA) because it provides a higher image quality.[26,27]

With the introduction of cholangioscopy, the diagnostic yield for malignancy in indeterminate biliary stricture has dramatically improved. On visualization, 4 cholangioscopic characteristics have been identified that are likely associated with malignancy such as tumor vessels, nodules, infiltrative lesions, and papillary projections.[28,29] These findings have been reported to have fair to a moderate interobserver agreement.[27,30,31] A 2020 systematic review and meta-analysis by Oliveira and colleagues reported a pooled sensitivity and specificity for the visual interpretation of biliary malignancies of 94% and 95%, respectively.[32] A large multicenter prospective case series published in 2020 reported a sensitivity of 86.7% and a specificity of 68.8% for the visual impression of malignancy.[33] Additionally, a study published in 2018 evaluating endoscopists' ability to diagnose or rule out malignancy based on 11 visual features that have been linked to malignancy reported that 6 features had at least moderate interobserver agreement (tubular, or branched/disorganized surface structures, adherent mucous, irregular margin, dark mucosa, and papillary projections). Moreover, this study reported that when endoscopists identified lesions as being benign or malignant, they were correct 89% and 83% of the time, respectively. When highly confident of a stricture being benign, they were correct in 96% of cases. When highly confident of a neoplasm, they were correct in 87% of the cases.[30] Certain characteristics can also be indicative of a benign process: smooth surface mucosa, a tapered and short luminal narrowing, and lack of neovascularization are features that likely indicate benign strictures.[28]

Although visual diagnosis has a high sensitivity, tissue diagnosis still presents a higher specificity and therefore remains the gold standard for diagnosis. The pillars of achieving tissue diagnosis are correctly targeting the stricture and tissue sample adequacy.[26] SOC allows targeted tissue collection under direct visualization with small forceps. Almadi and colleagues reported 75.3% sensitivity and 100% specificity with tissue sampling through SOC.[33] However, cholangioscopic sampling sensitivity, specificity, and accuracy have been reported to decrease in patients who had a previous ERCP with tissue sampling and brushing that were negative.[32] This could be due in part to previous tissue manipulation or simply because the stricture itself has characteristics that make a tissue diagnosis more challenging.

There are several variables that have been identified to decrease the sensitivity of cholangioscopy when working up indeterminate biliary strictures: personal history of primary sclerosing cholangitis, total serum bilirubin of greater than 3.2 mg/dL, prior biliary stent placement, hyperbilirubinemia, and endoscopists with less than 50 performed cholangioscopies.[34–36] Concern for cost is another one of the limiting factors for the availability of cholangioscopy. However, a study in Belgium showed that cholangioscopy can actually decrease the cost of evaluating indeterminate biliary strictures by reducing the number of total procedures performed to achieve a final diagnosis.[37]

In conclusion, cholangioscopy has proven to be a useful tool in the workup of indeterminate biliary strictures. Recent studies have shown that it consistently outperforms the sensitivity and specificity of ERCP in indeterminate biliary strictures..[11,27,37,38] Thus, it would be reasonable to perform cholangioscopy, if available, during the first ERCP to reduce the possibility of needing another ERCP if tissue diagnosis is inconclusive.[26]

Probe-based confocal laser endomicroscopy

Probe-based confocal laser endomicroscopy (pCLE) is an emerging technology that facilitates the direct visualization of the epithelium and up to 250 μm of the lamina propria using laser illumination.[39] It allows for an evaluation of cellular structures without the need for biopsy in patients undergoing ERCP. The confocal mini-probe is advanced through a duodenoscope into the biliary tree for its evaluation. The Paris criteria, a refinement of the Miami criteria, are used to interpret the imaging obtained by the pCLE.[40]

This technology has shown some utility in the differentiation between malignant and benign indeterminate biliary strictures.[41,42] It may also have substantial benefits in the evaluation of indeterminate biliary strictures because it has been recognized to have characteristics that exceed those of pathology.[17,43] A prospective multicenter international trial involving 112 patients reported that pCLE had a sensitivity of 89%, whereas tissue sampling alone had a sensitivity of 56% in diagnosing malignancy. However, pCLE was 72% percent specific, whereas tissue sampling was 100% specific.[44] Despite the promising results that this technology presents, it does not come without limitations. It is time-consuming, requires dedicated training for imaging interpretation, and needs fluorescein administration as a contrast agent. The interobserver agreement is suboptimal.[45] Additionally, it only allows for the evaluation of a small surface area at a time, and the up-front costs associated with capital equipment and probe purchasing may limit its availability to only a few centers.

Optical coherence tomography

Optical coherence tomography (OCT) is also a relatively new technology that uses infrared light to provide wide-field, in vivo cross-sectional imaging of the ductal wall. The 7 French balloon-style probe has an imaging depth of penetration up to 3 mm and a resolution of 7 μm, with a 6 cm scan length. It works similarly to pCLE, but it allows for a wider surface area evaluation which corrects one of the aforementioned limitations of pCLE. Like pCLE, certain OCT characteristics are suggestive of the underlying pathophysiology. A study published in 2018 reported that patients with cholangiocarcinoma were found to have thickening of the epithelium with projections, layering effacement, and a hyper-reflective surface with shadowing. Patients with PSC were characteristically found to have hyper-reflective subsurface structures with intact wall layering and onion skin layering. Additionally, patients with benign biliary strictures have been reported to show dilated hypo-reflective structures, clearly delineated epithelial layer, and clear layering in the inner mucosa.[46] The few clinical studies performed have shown promising results with sensitivities exceeding those of cytology and better specificity than pCLE when combined with brushings and biopsy.[46,47] The clinical impact of OCT in indeterminate biliary stricture evaluation is yet to be determined, but its use is limited by capital equipment and supply purchasing costs, a slight learning curve, and the fact that it does not allow tissue collection.

Intraductal ultrasound

Intraductal ultrasound (IDUS) is a widely used technology for bronchoscopy and can be used during ERCP to evaluate indeterminate biliary strictures. A mini-probe with radial cross-sectional imaging capability is inserted directly into the biliary lumen for evaluation. Although uncommonly performed, it has been reported to improve the yield in diagnosing indeterminate biliary strictures by providing high-resolution imaging of the biliary mural walls. It is capable of identifying masses, sessile tumors, and even adenopathy. A large cohort study with 397 patients reported that IDUS had 93% sensitivity and 89.5% specificity for identifying malignancy in patients with indeterminate biliary stricture.[48] Despite having high sensitivity and specificity, it is limited by its depth of penetration. Additionally, it does not allow biopsy samples to be collected like in EUS.[49]

Molecular studies

Biopsy samples acquired during ERCP have been shown to have a specificity as high as 100%, but have also been shown to have unacceptably low sensitivity. Molecular diagnostic tests have been shown to improve sensitivity.[15,50] Fluorescence in situ hybridization (FISH), which detects chromosomal abnormalities in the DNA, has had the greatest clinical impact. It has been studied as an individual test, but has been shown to provide a greater diagnostic value when used in combination with other diagnostic modalities.[51,52] A retrospective study that evaluated 281 patients over a 10-year period demonstrated that brush cytology in combination with FISH increased sensitivity from 35% to 54% without significantly affecting specificity. This study showed a further increase of sensitivity to 63% when brush cytology and FISH were combined with a 9p21 heterozygous or homozygous deletion.[15] Mutation profiling of KRAS or tumor suppressor gene mutations have also been reported to increase sensitivity in conjunction with FISH and cytology.[53,54] FISH has also proven to be particularly helpful in differentiating malignant cells in patients with primary sclerosing cholangitis in whom cytologic atypia is common due to chronic inflammation.[55]

Samples obtained by ERCP brushings can be assessed for KRAS oncogene mutation, tumor suppressor gene mutations, and loss of heterozygosity. These mutations can be evaluated on 10 genomic loci that have been shown to be associated with malignant strictures. These tests are convenient because they can be ordered after cytology has yielded a negative result and no additional ERCP is required. A study in 2019 showed that the sensitivity and specificity of tissue sampling by ERCP brushing could improve from 26% sensitivity with 100% specificity to 56% sensitivity with

97% specificity when adding mutation profiling to cytology alone.[53] Despite promising results, the clinical impact that these tests will have is yet to be determined.

SUMMARY

Indeterminate biliary strictures remain a diagnostic challenge. To date, there is no single tool or technique that can perfectly differentiate malignancy with both high specificity and sensitivity. At the cytology/molecular level, FISH, in combination with other molecular studies, has shown to be potentially helpful in differentiating benign and malignant pathology with specificities comparable to tissue pathology. At the interventional endoscopy level, cholangioscopy has become the diagnostic modality of choice for our practice in these complex cases and has the potential as a first-line tool for the endoscopic workup of indeterminate biliary strictures. Additional studies looking at the long-term outcomes and financial impact of early cholangioscopy for patients presenting with indeterminate biliary strictures are needed. Newer technologies such as pCLE, OCT, and IDUS are welcome additions to the diagnostic armamentarium with promising early study results. However, barriers to their use must be reduced before we can fully understand their utility in differentiating indeterminate biliary strictures.

CLINICS CARE POINTS

- For patients who present with indeterminate biliary strictures, cholangioscopy and EUS are extremely valuable in imaging and tissue diagnosis. Referral to a center that performs cholangioscopy and EUS routinely and has access to advanced cytology techniques like FISH is highly recommended.
- The decision to perform a surgical resection in a patient with an indeterminate biliary stricture should be multidisciplinary and involve both gastroenterology and surgery to ensure the patient is properly worked up and weighs the risks and benefits of the procedure. Referral to a high-volume tertiary care center with a multidisciplinary team may yield better outcomes for the patient.

DISCLOSURE

The authors have nothing to disclose.

REFERENCES

1. Singhi AD, Slivka A. Evaluation of indeterminate biliary strictures: is there life on MARS? Gastrointest Endosc 2020;92(2):320–2.
2. Singh A, Gelrud A, Agarwal B. Biliary strictures: diagnostic considerations and approach. Gastroenterol Rep (Oxf) 2015;3(1):22–31.
3. Parsa N, Khashab MA. The role of peroral cholangioscopy in evaluating indeterminate biliary strictures. Clin Endosc 2019;52(6):556–64.
4. Rana SS, Bhasin DK, Sharma V, et al. Role of endoscopic ultrasound in evaluation of unexplained common bile duct dilatation on magnetic resonance cholangiopancreatography. Ann Gastroenterol 2013;26(1):66–70.
5. Marrelli D, Caruso S, Pedrazzani C, et al. CA19-9 serum levels in obstructive jaundice: clinical value in benign and malignant conditions. Am J Surg 2009;198(3):333–9.

6. Giannini E, Borro P, Botta F, et al. Cholestasis is the main determinant of abnormal CA 19-9 levels in patients with liver cirrhosis. Int J Biol Markers 2000;15(3): 226–30.

7. Ferrone CR, Finkelstein DM, Thayer SP, et al. Perioperative CA19-9 levels can predict stage and survival in patients with resectable pancreatic adenocarcinoma. J Clin Oncol 2006;24(18):2897–902.

8. Mihmanli M, Dilege E, Demir U, et al. The use of tumor markers as predictors of prognosis in gastric cancer. Hepatogastroenterology 2004;51(59):1544–7.

9. Tsen A, Barbara M, Rosenkranz L. Dilemma of elevated CA 19-9 in biliary pathology. Pancreatology 2018;18(8):862–7.

10. Bowlus CL, Olson KA, Gershwin ME. Evaluation of indeterminate biliary strictures. Nat Rev Gastroenterol Hepatol 2016;13(1):28–37.

11. Sun B, Moon JH, Cai Q, et al. Review article: Asia-Pacific consensus recommendations on endoscopic tissue acquisition for biliary strictures. Aliment Pharmacol Ther 2018;48(2):138–51.

12. Topazian M. Endoscopic ultrasonography in the evaluation of indeterminate biliary strictures. Clin Endosc 2012;45(3):328–30.

13. Eloubeidi MA, Chen VK, Jhala NC, et al. Endoscopic ultrasound-guided fine needle aspiration biopsy of suspected cholangiocarcinoma. Clin Gastroenterol Hepatol 2004;2(3):209–13.

14. Mohamadnejad M, DeWitt JM, Sherman S, et al. Role of EUS for preoperative evaluation of cholangiocarcinoma: a large single-center experience. Gastrointest Endosc 2011;73(1):71–8.

15. Brooks C, Gausman V, Kokoy-Mondragon C, et al. Role of fluorescent in situ hybridization, cholangioscopic biopsies, and EUS-FNA in the evaluation of biliary strictures. Dig Dis Sci 2018;63(3):636–44.

16. Chiang A, Theriault M, Salim M, et al. The incremental benefit of EUS for the identification of malignancy in indeterminate extrahepatic biliary strictures: a systematic review and meta-analysis. Endoscopic ultrasound 2019;8(5):310–7.

17. American Society for Gastrointestinal Endoscopy Standards of Practice Committee, Anderson MA, Appalaneni V, et al. The role of endoscopy in the evaluation and treatment of patients with biliary neoplasia. Gastrointest Endosc 2013; 77(2):167–74.

18. Committee ASoP, Chathadi KV, Chandrasekhara V, et al. The role of ERCP in benign diseases of the biliary tract. Gastrointest Endosc 2015;81(4):795–803.

19. Korc P, Sherman S. ERCP tissue sampling. Gastrointest Endosc 2016;84(4): 557–71.

20. Navaneethan U, Njei B, Lourdusamy V, et al. Comparative effectiveness of biliary brush cytology and intraductal biopsy for detection of malignant biliary strictures: a systematic review and meta-analysis. Gastrointest Endosc 2015;81(1):168–76.

21. Fogel EL, deBellis M, McHenry L, et al. Effectiveness of a new long cytology brush in the evaluation of malignant biliary obstruction: a prospective study. Gastrointest Endosc 2006;63(1):71–7.

22. de Bellis M, Fogel EL, Sherman S, et al. Influence of stricture dilation and repeat brushing on the cancer detection rate of brush cytology in the evaluation of malignant biliary obstruction. Gastrointest Endosc 2003;58(2):176–82.

23. Fior-Gozlan M, Giovannini D, Rabeyrin M, et al. Monocentric study of bile aspiration associated with biliary brushing performed during endoscopic retrograde cholangiopancreatography in 239 patients with symptomatic biliary stricture. Cancer Cytopathol 2016;124(5):330–9.

24. Sugimoto S, Matsubayashi H, Kimura H, et al. Diagnosis of bile duct cancer by bile cytology: usefulness of post-brushing biliary lavage fluid. Endosc Int Open 2015;3(4):E323–8.

25. Fishman DS, Tarnasky PR, Patel SN, et al. Management of pancreaticobiliary disease using a new intra-ductal endoscope: the Texas experience. World J Gastroenterol 2009;15(11):1353–8.

26. Angsuwatcharakon P, Kulpatcharapong S, Moon JH, et al. Consensus guidelines on the role of cholangioscopy to diagnose indeterminate biliary stricture. HPB (Oxford) 2021. https://doi.org/10.1016/j.hpb.2021.05.005.

27. Kulpatcharapong S, Pittayanon R, Stephen JK, et al. Diagnostic performance of different cholangioscopes in patients with biliary strictures: a systematic review. Endoscopy 2020;52(3):174–85.

28. Seo DW, Lee SK, Yoo KS, et al. Cholangioscopic findings in bile duct tumors. Gastrointest Endosc 2000;52(5):630–4.

29. Kim HJ, Kim MH, Lee SK, et al. Tumor vessel: a valuable cholangioscopic clue of malignant biliary stricture. Gastrointest Endosc 2000;52(5):635–8.

30. Behary J, Keegan M, Craig PI. The interobserver agreement of optical features used to differentiate benign from neoplastic biliary lesions assessed at balloon-assisted cholangioscopy. J Gastroenterol Hepatol 2019;34(3):595–602.

31. Sethi A, Tyberg A, Slivka A, et al. Digital single-operator cholangioscopy (DSOC) improves interobserver agreement (IOA) and accuracy for evaluation of indeterminate biliary strictures: the Monaco classification. J Clin Gastroenterol 2020. https://doi.org/10.1097/MCG.0000000000001321.

32. de Oliveira P, de Moura DTH, Ribeiro IB, et al. Efficacy of digital single-operator cholangioscopy in the visual interpretation of indeterminate biliary strictures: a systematic review and meta-analysis. Surg Endosc 2020;34(8):3321–9.

33. Almadi MA, Itoi T, Moon JH, et al. Using single-operator cholangioscopy for endoscopic evaluation of indeterminate biliary strictures: results from a large multinational registry. Endoscopy 2020;52(7):574–82.

34. de Vries AB, van der Heide F, Ter Steege RWF, et al. Limited diagnostic accuracy and clinical impact of single-operator peroral cholangioscopy for indeterminate biliary strictures. Endoscopy 2020;52(2):107–14.

35. Njei B, McCarty TR, Varadarajulu S, et al. Systematic review with meta-analysis: endoscopic retrograde cholangiopancreatography-based modalities for the diagnosis of cholangiocarcinoma in primary sclerosing cholangitis. Aliment Pharmacol Ther 2016;44(11–12):1139–51.

36. Jang S, Stevens T, Kou L, et al. Efficacy of digital single-operator cholangioscopy and factors affecting its accuracy in the evaluation of indeterminate biliary stricture. Gastrointest Endosc 2020;91(2):385–93.e1.

37. Deprez PH, Garces Duran R, Moreels T, et al. The economic impact of using single-operator cholangioscopy for the treatment of difficult bile duct stones and diagnosis of indeterminate bile duct strictures. Endoscopy 2018;50(2):109–18.

38. Gerges C, Beyna T, Tang RSY, et al. Digital single-operator peroral cholangioscopy-guided biopsy sampling versus ERCP-guided brushing for indeterminate biliary strictures: a prospective, randomized, multicenter trial (with video). Gastrointest Endosc 2020;91(5):1105–13.

39. Othman MO, Wallace MB. Confocal laser endomicroscopy: is it prime time? J Clin Gastroenterol 2011;45(3):205–6.

40. Taunk P, Singh S, Lichtenstein D, et al. Improved classification of indeterminate biliary strictures by probe-based confocal laser endomicroscopy using the Paris Criteria following biliary stenting. J Gastroenterol Hepatol 2017;32(10):1778–83.

41. Loeser CS, Robert ME, Mennone A, et al. Confocal endomicroscopic examination of malignant biliary strictures and histologic correlation with lymphatics. J Clin Gastroenterol 2011;45(3):246–52.

42. Meining A, Frimberger E, Becker V, et al. Detection of cholangiocarcinoma in vivo using miniprobe-based confocal fluorescence microscopy. Clin Gastroenterol Hepatol 2008;6(9):1057–60.

43. Karia K, Kahaleh M. A review of probe-based confocal laser endomicroscopy for pancreaticobiliary disease. Clin Endosc 2016;49(5):462–6.

44. Slivka A, Gan I, Jamidar P, et al. Validation of the diagnostic accuracy of probe-based confocal laser endomicroscopy for the characterization of indeterminate biliary strictures: results of a prospective multicenter international study. Gastrointest Endosc 2015;81(2):282–90.

45. Talreja JP, Sethi A, Jamidar PA, et al. Interpretation of probe-based confocal laser endomicroscopy of indeterminate biliary strictures: is there any interobserver agreement? Dig Dis Sci 2012;57(12):3299–302.

46. Tyberg A, Xu MM, Gaidhane M, et al. Second generation optical coherence tomography: preliminary experience in pancreatic and biliary strictures. Dig Liver Dis 2018;50(11):1214–7.

47. Arvanitakis M, Hookey L, Tessier G, et al. Intraductal optical coherence tomography during endoscopic retrograde cholangiopancreatography for investigation of biliary strictures. Endoscopy 2009;41(8):696–701.

48. Meister T, Heinzow HS, Woestmeyer C, et al. Intraductal ultrasound substantiates diagnostics of bile duct strictures of uncertain etiology. World J Gastroenterol 2013;19(6):874–81.

49. Novikov A, Kowalski TE, Loren DE. Practical management of indeterminate biliary strictures. Gastrointest Endosc Clin North Am 2019;29(2):205–14.

50. Barr Fritcher EG, Voss JS, Jenkins SM, et al. Primary sclerosing cholangitis with equivocal cytology: fluorescence in situ hybridization and serum CA 19-9 predict risk of malignancy. Cancer Cytopathol 2013;121(12):708–17.

51. Smoczynski M, Jablonska A, Matyskiel A, et al. Routine brush cytology and fluorescence in situ hybridization for assessment of pancreatobiliary strictures. Gastrointest Endosc 2012;75(1):65–73.

52. Kipp BR, Stadheim LM, Halling SA, et al. A comparison of routine cytology and fluorescence in situ hybridization for the detection of malignant bile duct strictures. Am J Gastroenterol 2004;99(9):1675–81.

53. Kushnir VM, Mullady DK, Das K, et al. The diagnostic yield of malignancy comparing cytology, FISH, and molecular analysis of cell free cytology brush Supernatant in patients with biliary strictures undergoing endoscopic retrograde cholangiography (ERC): a prospective study. J Clin Gastroenterol 2019;53(9):686–92.

54. Gonda TA, Viterbo D, Gausman V, et al. Mutation profile and fluorescence in situ hybridization Analyses increase detection of malignancies in biliary strictures. Clin Gastroenterol Hepatol 2017;15(6):913–9.e11.

55. Quinn KP, Tabibian JH, Lindor KD. Clinical implications of serial versus isolated biliary fluorescence in situ hybridization (FISH) polysomy in primary sclerosing cholangitis. Scand J Gastroenterol 2017;52(4):377–81.

56. Choi SH, Han JK, Lee JM, et al. Differentiating malignant from benign common bile duct stricture with multiphasic helical CT. Radiology 2005;236(1):178–83.

57. Altman A, Zangan SM. Benign biliary strictures. Semin Intervent Radiol 2016; 33(4):297–306.
58. Soto JA, Alvarez O, Lopera JE, et al. Biliary obstruction: findings at MR cholangiography and cross-sectional MR imaging. Radiographics 2000;20(2):353–66.
59. Lee SS, Kim MH, Lee SK, et al. MR cholangiography versus cholangioscopy for evaluation of longitudinal extension of hilar cholangiocarcinoma. Gastrointest Endosc 2002;56(1):25–32.
60. Sadeghi A, Mohamadnejad M, Islami F, et al. Diagnostic yield of EUS-guided FNA for malignant biliary stricture: a systematic review and meta-analysis. Gastrointest Endosc 2016;83(2):290–8.e1.
61. Manta R, Frazzoni M, Conigliaro R, et al. SpyGlass single-operator peroral cholangioscopy in the evaluation of indeterminate biliary lesions: a single-center, prospective, cohort study. Surg Endosc 2013;27(5):1569–72.
62. Munot K, Raijman I, Khan V, et al. Aspiration fluid cytology during single operator cholangioscopy with targeted biopsy to improves the diagnostic yield in indeterminate biliary strictures. Diagn Cytopathol 2021;49(6):768–72.
63. Meining A, Chen YK, Pleskow D, et al. Direct visualization of indeterminate pancreaticobiliary strictures with probe-based confocal laser endomicroscopy: a multicenter experience. Gastrointest Endosc 2011;74(5):961–8.

Management of Biliary Complications in Liver Transplant Recipients

Justin J. Forde, MD, MS, Kalyan Ram Bhamidimarri, MD, MPH*

KEYWORDS

- Liver transplantation • Biliary complications • Endoscopic intervention • ERCP
- Biliary stricture

KEY POINTS

- Biliary complications are considered the Achilles' heel of liver transplantation (LT) and are encountered in up to a quarter of the patients following LT.
- Risk factors for biliary complications include graft factors (donation after cardiac death (DCD), living donor liver transplant (LDLT)), surgical factors (prolonged ischemia time, duct mismatch, or trauma), donor factors (cytomegalovirus (CMV) infection, ABO blood group mismatch), vascular factors (hepatic artery thrombosis (HAT) or stenosis), or recipient factors (undiagnosed primary sclerosing cholangitis (PSC), aberrant vascular anatomy, or hypercoagulable state).
- Signs and symptoms of biliary complications can be mild or significantly deranged in liver transplant recipients due to altered anatomy and immunosuppression. Therefore, a high index of clinical suspicion is required for early diagnosis and management.
- Abnormal liver biochemistry with features of cholestasis should trigger the evaluation for biliopathy with abdominal ultrasound and Doppler to evaluate the hepatic vasculature and biliary tree. Subsequent strategies could include computed tomography (CT) scan or magnetic resonance imaging/cholangiopancreatography (MRI/MRCP).
- Obvious bile duct pathology with a normal hepatic artery should be managed endoscopically with endoscopic retrograde cholangiopancreatography (ERCP) if feasible, though patients with altered anatomy may require percutaneous intervention. Surgical intervention is reserved if endoscopic or percutaneous modalities are not effective or feasible.

INTRODUCTION

Liver transplantation (LT) is the only curative option for patients with acute liver failure and end-stage liver disease.[1] Initial outcomes with LT since its inception in the 1960s were dismal due to significant challenges in the restoration of bilio-enteric continuity.[2] Refinements in surgical techniques and advances in perioperative care and immunosuppression have led to significant improvements in outcomes in recent decades.[2]

Division of Digestive Health and Liver Diseases, University of Miami Miller School of Medicine, 1295 Northwest 14th Street, Suite A, Miami, FL 33136, USA
* Corresponding author.
E-mail address: KBhamidimarri@med.miami.edu

Clin Liver Dis 26 (2022) 81–99
https://doi.org/10.1016/j.cld.2021.08.008
1089-3261/22/© 2021 Elsevier Inc. All rights reserved.

Currently, the 1-year patient survival following LT exceeds 85%.[3,4] Despite this, biliary complications remain a major source of morbidity and mortality after LT with a reported incidence of 10% to 25% than early accounts which cite an incidence of up to 50%.[1,3,5] Common biliary complications following liver transplant include biliary strictures, bile leaks, bile duct stones, and sphincter of Oddi dysfunction.[6] Risk factors include hepatic artery thrombosis (HAT), perioperative bleeding, ischemia, and or reperfusion injury, immunologic from acute cellular rejection, infectious etiologies such as cytomegalovirus (CMV), t-tube or stent-related complications, and technical failure from surgical technique and mismatch between the size of donor and recipient bile duct.[7] Considerable variation occurs in the clinical presentation of postliver transplant biliary complications and early diagnosis may be challenging due to the subtle or mild onset of symptoms. Magnetic resonance imaging (MRI), a noninvasive method, has significantly changed our diagnostic approach in evaluating biliary disorders.[8] The preferred treatment approach can vary based on the complication and anatomy; however, endoscopic or percutaneous approaches are often preferable and more invasive surgical techniques are reserved for refractory conditions. In the following article, we will outline the evaluation and management of biliary complications in liver transplant recipients.

PATHOPHYSIOLOGY AND RISK FACTORS

The mechanisms of biliary injury and subsequent biliary complications following LT vary and are often related to decreased wound healing secondary to immunosuppression, immunologic injury from CMV infection, preservation injury secondary to ischemia, altered anatomy, and issues from surgical technique.[1,9] Many complications are related to the tenuous nature of the blood supply to the bile ducts, which is derived solely from vessels originating from the hepatic artery. Interruptions in hepatic artery blood supply can lead to irreversible damage to the intra and extrahepatic bile ducts and lead to complications such as complex stricture formation. Devascularization of the ducts can occur due to technical factors such as failure to recognize anomalous anatomy of the biliary tree during organ procurement or transplantation, technically challenging reconstruction due to the duct size or the presence of multiple ducts.[10] HAT, acute rejection, and CMV infection are also significant causes of decreased perfusion of the biliary tree. Necrosis of the bile ducts can occur from this impaired blood flow resulting in bile leaks and bilomas. Bile leaks, which can occur particularly in the case of partial LT, are recognized as an independent risk factor for the development of anastomotic strictures (ASs).[11] Stricture formation can lead to relative biliary stasis and sloughing of the biliary lining which can lead to intraductal filling defects such as casts, sludge, and stones. These obstructive processes further contribute to bile leaks and bilomas.

Surgical Technique and Anastomosis Type

Several factors have been identified as contributing to increased risk for developing biliary complications after LT (**Table 1**). Factors relating to biliary anastomosis such as surgical technique especially pose significant risk and are often the cause of early complications such as bile leaks and strictures. These factors include suture-related insufficiencies, inappropriate suture material or excessive tension at the anastomosis, excessive use of electrocauterization for bleeding, and biliary reconstruction type.[12] The 2 most common types of biliary reconstruction are choledocho-choledochostomy (CC) and choledochojejunostomy (CJ) with Roux-en-Y loop. It is generally accepted that the rate of complications is similar between techniques; however, there is evidence to suggest

Table 1 Risk factors associated with biliary complications	
Risk Factors	**Associated Complication**
Donor Characteristics (Deceased donor graft, Living Donor, Older donor)	• Non-anastomotic strictures • Stones, sludge, casts, clots • Hepatic artery thrombosis • Bile leaks (LDLT)
Graft Characteristics (Steatosis, increased cold, and warm ischemia times)	• Non-anastomotic • Anastomotic strictures • Stones, sludge, casts, clots • Bile leaks
Vascular (hepatic artery thrombosis, stenosis, strictures)	• Bile leaks • Anastomotic stricture • Non-anastomotic stricture • Anastomotic disruption • Biliary casts
Anastomosis type (duct-to-duct choledochocholedochostomy vs Roux-en-y choledochojejunostomy)	• Theoretically duct-to-duct choledocho-choledochostomy prevents enteric reflux and decreases the risk of cholangitis though data are conflicting
Surgical Technique (Excessive electrocautery or dissection, tension on the biliary anastomosis, inappropriate suture material, t-tube insertion)	• Anastomotic strictures • Bile leaks • Sphincter of Oddi dysfunction
Infectious (Cytomegalovirus, intraabdominal infections, viral hepatitis recurrence)	• Anastomotic strictures • Non-anastomotic strictures • Cholangitis or peritonitis

that there is a slightly increased risk of bacterial colonization, bleeding, and leaks with Roux-en-Y.[13,14] There are no guidelines that dictate the optimal type of suture material, suture type, or anastomosis that should be performed and often the decision is based on factors such as surgeon preference, anatomy, etiology of the underlying liver disease, and prior surgeries of the biliary system. CC reconstruction is preferred and approximately three-quarters of cadaveric orthotopic liver transplants in adults are performed in this manner.[15,16] The main advantages of duct-to-duct anastomosis include that it is technically easier and that it spares the sphincter of Oddi that maintains the natural reflux barrier to enteric contents into the biliary tree and decreases the risk of cholangitis.[15] CC can be performed with end-to-end anastomosis or side to side, with no difference in biliary complications between the 2 in the absence of T-tube placement.[17,18] Although CC is often preferred, it may not be feasible in instances of biliary atresia or duct size mismatch.[15] Roux-en-Y has been the preferred biliary reconstruction in LT for primary sclerosing cholangitis (PSC) due to concerns for possible cholangiocarcinoma arising from the duct remnant; however, outcomes between the 2 reconstruction types are similar with regard to the rates of complications, recurrent PSC, or graft survival.[19]

T-Tubes

T-tubes were routinely placed during LT in the past to bridge the anastomosis, allow postoperative assessment of bile quality, and for direct radiographic access to the biliary tree. In some studies, T-tube placement has been observed to potentially reduce the incidence of AS formation following LT.[18] Despite this, comparative studies have shown an increased incidence of complications such strictures, leaks, and cholangitis with their use making their routine placement controversial.[15,20,21] Few randomized controlled trials (RCTs) evaluating this have been performed and those available have had somewhat conflicting results.[22,23] Notably, most early bile leaks after LT are seen at the T-Tube insertion site and other complications have been reported in 33% of T-tube removals.[24,25] T-tubes have also been observed to be less cost-effective with longer length of stay, increased need for radiological studies, and overall greater use of hospital resources.[26] Due to the overall increased risk of complications, the usage of T-tube has declined across all transplant centers since the 1990s.[1] Alternatively, utilization of indwelling transcystic stents has been proposed to secure the biliary anastomosis and allow for cholangiography with the benefit of earlier withdrawal time and less biliary complications than T-tubes.[27] Complications such as obstruction, migration, erosion, and hemobilia were still observed.

Vascular Complications

HAT is a rare and potentially catastrophic complication that can occur after LT.[28] Although overall rare, HAT is the most common vascular complication following LT seen both early and late.[29] Overall risk factors associated with HAT include surgical issues relating to the anastomosis, increased donor age (>60), extended cold ischemia time, ABO incompatibility, cigarette smoking, CMV-negative recipient, rejection, and PSC.[12,30] HAT is the most common cause of biliary strictures in the posttransplant period, but is also associated with biliary ischemia, necrosis, sepsis, hepatic insufficiency, and graft loss and should be suspected when there is any biliary complication.[31] The actual incidence of early HAT is unknown; however, in large liver transplant centers, it has been observed to be 3%. HAT is the culprit in almost 50% of patients with non-anastomotic biliary strictures.[32] HAT is associated with increased requirements for interventions and poorer outcomes following interventions. Biliary complications from arterial insufficiency have been observed to require intervention in 45% than 22% without arterial complications.[10] Endoscopic intervention for anastomotic biliary strictures caused by HAT resulted in a 1-year cumulative primary patency rate of 0%, whereas patients with patent hepatic artery had a success rate of 45%.[33] Doppler ultrasound is the gold standard modality for assessing the patency of the hepatic artery.[29] Subsequent angiography can be used to confirm the diagnosis when ultrasound is suggestive, but inconclusive.[34] Management options for HAT vary based on the acuity of the thrombosis and patient condition. In acute HAT, surgical or endovascular revascularization versus retransplantation must be considered. Although historically retransplantation was preferred as it provided the best survival, the supply of donor livers is prohibitive and endovascular management is, therefore, preferred to rescue the graft when plausible.[35] Open surgical revascularization can also be attempted with an approach that is based on the state of the arterial stump of the graft and recipient.[35] In a minority of cases of late HAT with slow arterial occlusion, no intervention is needed as patients will develop collateral circulation.[29,36] Retransplant should be performed in symptomatic patients with severe allotransplant dysfunction.

Although HAT is the most common cause of biliary strictures, 1.4% of all deceased-donor orthotopic liver transplants (OLTs) with biliary strictures present without any obvious vascular impairment.[35] When these strictures resemble biliary tract changes seen in patients with ischemic damage to the biliary tree they are referred to as ischemic-type biliary lesions (ITBLs). These lesions have been described in increased frequency in patients with cold ischemia times of greater than 10 to 12 hours or delayed arterialization of the graft. Other vascular risk factors include prior existing splenic artery steal syndrome, arteriosclerotic stenosis of the celiac axis, or intermittent stenosis of the celiac axis during inspiration by the arcuate ligament.[37]

Other Factors

CMV is the most common viral pathogen in patients receiving OLT with potential involvement of the liver, gastrointestinal tract, lung, or systemic infection.[38] Biliary complications after LT have been demonstrated more commonly in individuals with CMV viremia and in patients with LT with primary CMV infection.[39] Additionally, infection can result in acute cholestatic hepatitis in this immunocompromised population.[40] Although routine prophylaxis of seronegative recipients has resulted in decreased risk, CMV infection remains a risk factor for biliary complications, graft loss, and mortality after LT.[39,41] The proposed pathophysiology involves the precipitation of chronic rejection by CMV-induced human leukocyte antigen expression in transplant recipients.[42]

CLINICAL PRESENTATION AND DIAGNOSIS OF BILIARY COMPLICATIONS
Clinical Presentation

Due to altered anatomy, immunosuppression, denervation of biliary structures transplanted patients may often present differently than patients who have not had LT. Patients may present with asymptomatic elevation in serum chemical markers or with nonspecific symptoms such as fever, right upper quadrant pain, anorexia, abdominal distension, right-shoulder pain, ileus, or sustained output through drain sites.[43,44] Others present with biliary peritonitis or stigmata of septic shock from ascending cholangitis, bilomas, and bile leaks.[44] A high index of suspicion is required to diagnose biliary complications early in LT recipients with vague symptoms or elevations in serum aminotransferases, bilirubin, alkaline phosphatase, and or gamma-glutamyl transferase (GGT).

Diagnostic Imaging

The initial assessment usually begins with laboratory evaluation and abdominal imaging with transabdominal Doppler ultrasound. Ultrasound is a preferred initial imaging modality as it is a relatively inexpensive and noninvasive modality that allows for the evaluation of the biliary tree, liver parenchyma, perihepatic fluid collections, and flow characteristics of the hepatic vasculature. Of note in the presence of dilated bile ducts the positive predictive value of ultrasound is high; however, sensitivity is only 38% to 68% in the absence of biliary ductal dilation.[45,46] Further workup with more sensitive techniques should be pursued in the absence of bile duct dilation on ultrasonography. Computed tomography angiography (CTA) or hepatic angiography may be helpful if there is a suggestion of hepatic artery thrombus or stenosis on initial ultrasound and should be the next step in evaluation. Endoscopic ultrasound (EUS) has recently become a viable diagnostic modality with the ability for Doppler assessment.

If initial imaging is negative and suspicion for biliary complications remains high, cholangiography is the reference standard for diagnosis and should be obtained.[43,47] Magnetic resonance imaging has high sensitivity for the diagnosis of biliary strictures (93%–100%) and stones (90%–95%).[48,49] Contraindications that may preclude the use of MRCP include nonremovable metallic foreign bodies, claustrophobia, and impaired renal function. The decision to pursue either endoscopic or percutaneous intervention is based on patient anatomy, presence or absence of biliary ductal dilation, and patient clinical condition.

Graft Biopsy

Of note, graft biopsy is frequently pursued before cholangiopathy to evaluate for possible rejection, ischemia, or other pathology. Biopsy has been found to have a sensitivity of 87% and specificity of 87% for the diagnosis of biliary complications (than imaging as the gold standard).[50] It is important to note that histologic features of extrahepatic bile duct obstruction such as portal inflammation may be misinterpreted as rejection or hepatitis C infection.[50,51]

MANAGEMENT

In the past biliary complications following LT were managed with surgical revisions, which were invasive and posed an increased risk of complications. With the evolution of endoscopic treatments, endoscopic retrograde cholangiopancreatography (ERCP) has become the standard therapy when feasible. Endoscopic interventions are generally safe following LT with complications reported in 6%–10% of patients, which is similar to nontransplant patients.[52,53] The most common complications include pancreatitis, cholangitis, and postsphincterotomy bleeding.[54] Other, less common complications include perforation, bile leak, subcapsular hematoma, and stent migration.[55]

Bile Leaks

Bile leaks are most frequently encountered within the first 1 to 3 months following LT commonly at the anastomotic site, exit site of the T-tube, or at the cystic duct remnant.[15,56] Bile leaks are observed following 2% to 25% of liver transplants and the etiology somewhat differs based on the location of the leak.[43,56] Risk factors for early bile leaks include insufficient perfusion from the hepatic artery or other technical factors involved with the transplantation. Late bile duct leaks usually occur following the removal of the T-tube and are often related to inadequate maturation of the T-tube tract due to immunosuppression. Leaks at the anastomosis usually occur early and are frequently caused by ischemic necrosis, downstream obstruction, hypertension of the Sphincter of Oddi, or T-tube removal.[11] Anastomotic leaks are most common and they are accompanied by biliary strictures in 26% of cases.[11] Nonanastomotic leaks more frequently occur because of vascular insufficiency following HAT or T-tube removal.[25,57] Leaks should be suspected in patients who have pain following T-tube removal, present with stigmata of peritonitis, and in patients who have fluid collections observed on imaging studies. In patients with T-tubes, the diagnosis can be made with a T-tube cholangiogram versus ERCP. Hepatobiliary scintigraphy (HIDA) scan can aid in making the diagnosis when there is low suspicion for leak and has a sensitivity of approximately 50% and a specificity of approximately 80%.[58,59]

Asymptomatic patients with small leaks may not require intervention and are sometimes managed conservatively. Therapeutic options for significant leaks include repeat surgical intervention, percutaneous transhepatic biliary drainage (PTBD), and endoscopic methodologies such as ERCP. All bile leaks occurring after duct-to-duct anastomosis, with rare exceptions, can be managed endoscopically.[60] The overall endoscopic approach to the treatment of postoperative bile leaks is the diversion of bile and reduction of the transpapillary pressure and facilitate closure. Endoscopic stent placement with or without sphincterotomy essentially reduces the transpapillary gradient to zero permitting the effective diversion of bile. Although there are no guidelines on optimal endoscopic intervention for the management of bile leaks, ERCP with stent placement has been shown to be more effective than sphincterotomy alone.[60] This tactic is successful in up to 90% of early leaks, which will typically resolve within 5 weeks.[61,62] Due to delayed healing in the setting of immunosuppression following LT, stents for bile leaks following transplantation are generally kept in place for approximately 2 months versus 4 to 6 weeks as in postcholecystectomy leaks.[63] Stents are usually not replaced unless there is evidence of obstruction and there is no further indication for prolonged stenting once the leak has resolved. In the case of small anastomotic leaks whereby a T-tube is present management is often successful with simply leaving the tube open.[58] Endoscopic naso-biliary catheter placement allows for the close monitoring of closure and is advantageous in that it can be removed without the need for a repeat endoscopic procedure.[64] Disadvantages include patient tolerance and potential for the inadvertent dislodgement of the tube. Additionally, with the diversion of bile outside of the body, the levels of immunosuppressive agents (such as cyclosporine) must be monitored carefully as they may decline in the absence of enterohepatic circulation.[64] Anastomotic leaks in patients with Roux-en-Y reconstruction are somewhat less common and PTBD must be considered in this population when the biliary orifice cannot be reached or whereby enteroscopy-assisted ERCP is not available. Percutaneous transhepatic cholangiogram (PTC) can be challenging in biliary leaks due to the decompression of the biliary tree and subsequent small duct size which are difficult to target. Surgery may be required for a bile leak associated with severe abdominal sepsis, disruption of the biliary anastomosis, bile duct necrosis, or failure of endoscopic or percutaneous management strategies.

Cut surface leaks often originate from bile ducts that are transected during liver biopsy or during resection in living donor transplants may take up to 8 weeks to resolve the following intervention. Overall, the evidence suggests a resolution of 85% to 100% of bile leaks with the above modalities.[65] Of note bile leaks that form because of ischemia are often a challenge as they usually do not respond to nonoperative diversion of biliary flow.[34]

Rupture of the biliary ducts may occur due to bile duct necrosis secondary to HAT resulting in bile spillage into the hepatic parenchyma or abdominal cavity resulting in bilomas.[47] Most bilomas will occur in the perihepatic area outside of the hepatic parenchyma. A minority of bilomas occur inside of the parenchyma of the liver and in communication with the biliary tree.[64] If small these bilomas may resolve spontaneously without treatment though they are sometimes managed endoscopically with transpapillary stent placement.[66,67] Generally, bilomas that are large and not in communication with the bile ducts are managed with antibiotics and percutaneous drainage as they have a significant risk of infection. Surgical drainage is usually reserved as a last option in refractory bile leaks that are not adequately controlled with nonsurgical modalities.[68]

Hemobilia

Hemobilia is a relatively rare complication seen after OLT that is usually associated with liver biopsy or PTC. The classic presentation includes right upper quadrant abdominal pain, jaundice, and gastrointestinal bleeding; however, this is not a common presentation. Hemobilia can result in biliary obstruction due to the formation of intraductal blood clots. The mainstay of treatment involved hemostasis and clearance of biliary obstruction resulting from clots with ERCP. In most cases, bleeding is self-limited and only requires conservative management including the correction of coagulopathy if present. In cases whereby bleeding does not spontaneously resolve, interventional radiology embolization may be required.[43,62]

Biliary Strictures

Biliary strictures are the most commonly encountered complication after LT and are encountered as of late complications following LT, most commonly 5 to 8 months after transplantation.[15] They are seen in 5% to 15% of deceased donor transplants, 28%–32% of living donor transplants, and account for approximately 40% of all biliary complications after LT.[15,44,69] They are characterized as ASs or non–ASs.

Anastomotic strictures

ASs are defined as isolated strictures occurring within 5 mm of the duct-to-duct anastomosis. They are typically single, short, and localized to the anastomosis site with an incidence of 4% to 9% following all LT (**Fig. 1**).[11] Most AS occur within the first 12 months following an LT; however, they have been observed up to 11 years post-transplant.[61] Early AS, occurring within 3 weeks, are likely due to narrowing from surgery such as inadequate mucosa to mucosa anastomosis and narrowing due to edematous pressure.[11] Bile leaks early in the postoperative course are a risk factor for early AS formation, possibly secondary to the inflammatory effect of bile. Late strictures are thought to occur from the fibrosis that results from local ischemia.[70] Additional risk factors for AS include older donor, male to female mismatch, prolonged warm and cold ischemia time, Roux-en-Y reconstruction, and the graft used for transplantation. Graft type is cited as the most important risk factor in AS formation with a significant risk being associated with the use of grafts from living-related donors and use of split liver, likely from size mismatch inherent to these transplantation types.[11,71] Patients may present with abdominal pain, fever, and jaundice or have asymptomatic cholestasis on chemistries. Imaging may demonstrate the dilation of the biliary tree proximal to the biliary anastomosis.

Clinically significant AS require intervention, preferably endoscopic management involving ERCP with sphincterotomy, balloon dilation, and placement of plastic stents. Balloon dilation without stenting has been evaluated and is associated with a higher rate of recurrent stricture versus dilation and stenting.[72] The characteristic appearance of cholangiography is a thin narrowing at the biliary anastomosis. AS identified within 2 to 4 months after LT generally have a good response to ERCP with sphincterotomy and 3 to 6 months of stenting which may resolve the stricture without further interventions.[11] More commonly biliary stents are exchanged at intervals of 3 months to avoid stent occlusion and bacterial cholangitis. During exchanges, the previously placed stent is removed, the stricture is dilated, and a new stent or stents are placed across the stricture to increase the diameter of the stricture (**Fig. 2**).[73] Success rates of 70%–100% have been reported in stricture resolution in patients undergoing serial procedures.[11,73,74] Percutaneous intervention with PTC may be required in the setting of Roux-en-Y reconstruction due to inability to reach the biliary orifice with the endoscope or in cases of failure to traverse an AS with the guidewire during ERCP. Surgical revision may be required in stable patients with AS that is, difficult to treat endoscopically or percutaneously.

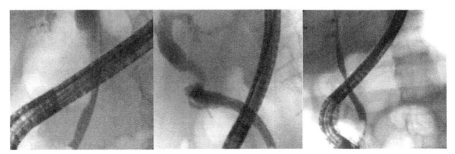

Fig. 1. Fluoroscopic images showing biliary anastomotic stricture.

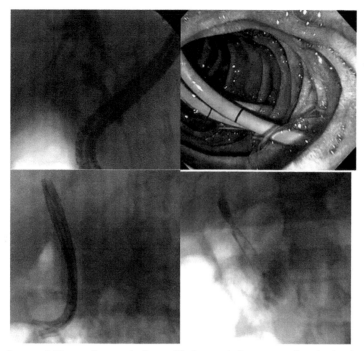

Fig. 2. Refractory biliary strictures: balloon dilation and placement of multiple plastic stents or self-expandable metallic stent.

Patients with initial presentation that is, delayed (>6) months or associated with very tight strictures require lifelong surveillance for stricture recurrence. This surveillance should be tailored and may include periodic evaluation of liver enzymes, ultrasound, or MRCP depending on the characteristics of the initial stricture.

Non-anastomotic strictures

Non–ASs are irregularities in the biliary tree located greater than 1 cm from the surgical anastomosis in a patient with a patent hepatic artery. Non-anastomotic strictures (NAS) are commonly thought to be ischemic type strictures arising from impaired blood flow or less commonly secondary to recurrence of an underlying disease process.[11] Compared with AS they are usually multiple, longer, and found in the hilar region or diffusely intrahepatic in the donor duct proximal to the anastomosis site.[11] NAS incidence ranges from 5% to 15% occurring at a mean time of 3.3 to 5.9-months post–OLT.[21,75] Nonischemic etiologies leading to NAS include immunologic as in ABO-incompatible grafts, patients with autoimmune hepatitis, PSC, and chronic ductopenic rejection. The presentation in NAS is similar to that of AS though NAS are typically more difficult to manage and result in poorer outcomes.[76] Those with HAT require urgent revascularization or early retransplantation. Endoscopic or percutaneous interventions are recommended for those without thrombosis. Multiple strictures may be seen which causes a cholangiographic appearance similar to PSC. These strictures may lead to the retention of sludge and cast formation, predisposing the patient to episodes of cholangitis. Successful intervention depends largely on factors such as the location, number, and severity of the strictured area. Endoscopic intervention usually consists of ERCP with dilation using 4–6 mm balloon than 6–8 mm balloon as used for AS with subsequent sphincterotomy and placement of 10 to 11.5 Fr plastic stents. As with AS, these stents are typically replaced every 3 months. Time to response is known to be more prolonged than with AS with a median time of 185 days for NAS versus 67 days for AS in an illustrative study.[76] The outcomes are less favorable for NAS with only 50% of patients having a long-term response with endoscopic dilation and stenting.[47,77] Up to 50% of patients will require retransplantation or die from complications associated with NAS. Generally, the presence of multiple strictures is associated with poor graft survival and requires retransplantation.[78]

Sphincter of Oddi Dysfunction

Sphincter of Oddi dysfunction (SOD) following OLT is estimated to occur at an incidence of 2%–5% and is commonly referred to as papillary dyskinesia, biliary spasm, papillary stenosis, or ampullary dysfunction.[43,47] These terms have been used to describe the biliary or pancreatic obstruction relating to mechanical or functional abnormalities of the sphincter of Oddi. Data suggest that these structural and functional disorders as defined by the Rome IV criteria (**Box 1**) are rare after LT.[79] SOD with increased basal pressure of the sphincter can lead to the dilation of the recipient and donor bile duct with biochemical abnormalities. SOD is thought to be due to the denervation of the sphincter during OLT or stenosis from chronic inflammation and resultant fibrosis.[15] The diagnosis is suspected in patients with cholestasis and uniform dilation of the bile ducts in the absence of evidence of obstruction on imaging. Biliary manometry can be used to confirm the diagnosis. The goals of treatment for symptomatic patients with sphincter of Oddi dysfunction are to reduce or eliminate pain and to improve the flow of bile into the duodenum. Although there are no evidence-based recommendations for management, ERCP with sphincterotomy with or without stenting is an acceptable option. During ERCP the biliary or pancreatic segment of the sphincter of Oddi can be cut with electrocautery, which has been associated with improvement or elimination of pain in up to 83% of patients.[80] The clinical course is largely unpredictable after intervention and results are widely variable. Pharmacologic treatment with drugs such as calcium channel blockers and nitrates may provide benefits in patients who are high risk for endoscopic management with ERCP.

BILIARY STONES, SLUDGE, AND CASTS

Common bile duct filling defects can occur due to biliary stones, sludge, blood clots, casts, and or mispositioned stents. Bile duct obstruction from stones or sludge can occur following LT. Stones and sludge can result from any process that leads to increased viscosity or decreased flow of bile. This is often seen in the setting of biliary

---

Box 1
Rome criteria

Rome IV Criteria for sphincter of Oddi dysfunction
- Criteria for biliary pain are met
  - Pain in the epigastrium or RUQ
  - Episodes ≥30 minutes
  - Recurrent symptoms at different intervals
  - Pain builds to a steady level.
  - Pain is severe.
  - Pain is not significantly associated with bowel movements.
  - Pain is not significantly related to postural change or acid suppression.
- Absence of bile duct stones or other structural abnormalities
- Elevated liver enzymes or dilated bile duct, but not both

stricture in the posttransplant recipients. However, warm and cold ischemia, bacterial infections, and obstructions also can predispose to stone formation.[43,81,82] There is also limited evidence to support that cyclosporine may cause stone formation through the inhibition of bile secretion.[83] Stones are often seen as a late complication following LT, at a median of 19 months.[47] Biliary casts form from the sloughing of the mucosa due to damage from ischemia, obstruction, or infection.[81] Patients who develop biliary obstruction from biliary casts have poor graft survival and worse post–LT outcomes. Often patients present with abdominal pain, cholestasis and less often, cholangitis. Abdominal ultrasound or CT scans are often the first step in assessment; however, cholangiography is the only reliable imaging modality to detect sludge. Stones, sludge, and casts are seen as filling defects during MRCP or ERCP. Management involves ERCP with a combination of techniques including sphincterotomy, lithotripsy, stent placement, and balloon and basket extraction (**Fig. 3**). Despite highly effective techniques for endoscopic stone extraction factors such as stone size, impacted stones, or stones lodged behind strictures may lead to treatment failure. Patients with Roux-en-Y CJ often require percutaneous intervention.

COMPLICATIONS FOLLOWING LIVING DONOR TRANSPLANTATION

Overall living donor transplants provide significant benefits including lower overall costs, better graft availability, reduced cold ischemia time, and lower incidence of steroid-resistant rejection.[84,85] Biliary complications are, however, more common following living donor LT than deceased donor transplants with an overall incidence of 6%–40%.[86,87] These complications often present within few weeks or within months of transplantation. The etiologies for this increased incidence are numerous and risk factors include reconstruction type, recipient age and sex, ABO blood type incompatibility, original disease process, CMV infection, and use of multiple ducts for anastomosis.[88] Two-thirds of biliary complications following living donor transplantation were identified as bile leaks than one-third in deceased donor transplants with an overall incidence of 6% to 27%.[89,90] These bile leaks frequently occur at the location of the cut surface of the liver and less commonly at the anastomosis. Biliary strictures are also commonly encountered following living donor liver transplant (LDLT) with an incidence of 13% to 21%.[86,89] These

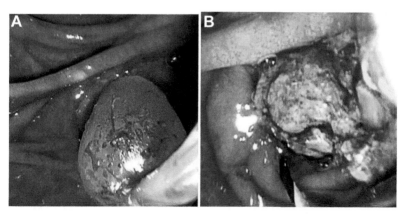

Fig. 3. Endoscopic management of filling defects (A). Endoscopic image showing sphincteroplasty with dilation balloon (B). Endoscopic image showing biliary stone extraction using extractor balloon.

strictures may be anastomotic or non-anastomotic as with deceased donor transplants. Their pathophysiology is related to predominantly operative factors such as biliary ischemia, cold ischemia time, and anastomosis type in the case of ASs and ischemia or autoimmune injury in the case of non–ASs.[12] Donors may also experience biliary complications such as leaks and strictures, the incidence of which has been observed in 0.4% to 13% of donors.[91] These complications are most often seen following right lobe donations. Evaluation and management of these complications is the same as with recipients.

ADVANCED ENDOSCOPIC TECHNIQUES
Digital Cholangioscopy

In the last decade, innovations in endoscopic devices and techniques have provided enhanced options for the evaluation and management of biliary complications following LT. Cholangioscopy involves the direct visualization of the biliary and pancreatic ducts through miniature endoscopes which are passed through the working channel of a duodenoscope during ERCP. Early cholangioscopy techniques required 2 experienced endoscopists, were low definition, and were high cost which limited their use. The advent of the high-definition single operator per oral cholangioscopy (SOC) system (SpyGlass [Boston Scientific Corp, Massachusetts, USA]) has provided a useful adjunct to ERCP (**Fig. 4**).[92] Although the technique has several useful applications, it is frequently used for the investigation of indeterminate biliary strictures or for the removal of difficult stones. SOC has been shown to provide improved visualization of strictures and superior detection of stones and biliary casts as it overcomes the issue of dense contrast media masking these filling defects.[92] SOC-guided electrohydraulic lithotripsy allows for the fragmentation and removal of stones that are not amenable to more conventional endoscopic removal techniques due to their size, location, or patient anatomy. This is preferred extracorporeal shock wave lithotripsy (ESWL) as it has similar or improved stone clearance, ESWL still requires subsequent ERCP for fragment removal, and that it obviates coordination with urology which is frequently needed with ESWL.[93]

Enteroscopy

Due to inability to reach the biliary orifice, ERCP has high failure rates in patients with Roux-en-Y reconstruction making it necessary to consider alternatives such as PTC. In high-volume centers with experienced endoscopists, ERCP is often successfully performed even in patients with Roux-en-Y in this population using a variable stiffness

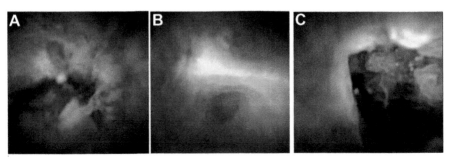

Fig. 4. Spyglass (*A, B*). Cholangioscopy demonstrating biliary strictures (*C*). cholangioscopy demonstrating hilar malignancy.

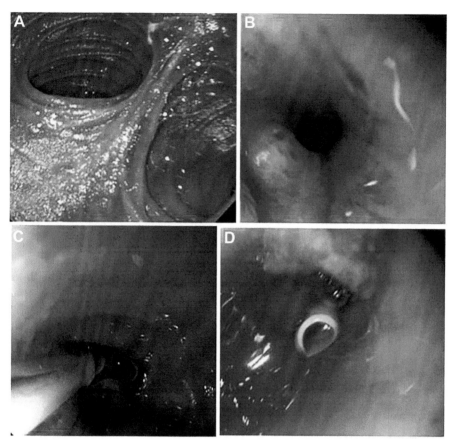

Fig. 5. Single balloon enteroscopy-assisted ERCP in LT recipients with hepaticojejunostomy (*A*). Roux-en-Y entero-enteric anastomosis (*B*). Biliary orifice Roux en Y limb (*C*). Insertion of long extractor balloon (*D*). SBE-assisted stent insertion.

pediatric colonoscope or with balloon-assisted deep small bowel enteroscopy techniques (**Fig. 5**).[94]

Endoscopic Ultrasound

EUS is increasingly being used for the evaluation of biliary complications post–LT given its high sensitivity (94.6%).[95] Interventional EUS techniques such as EUS-guided transgastric drainage of bilomas or liver biopsies provide alternatives to percutaneous approaches. Formation of EUS-guided gastrostomy followed by ERCP performed through the gastrostomy port provides additional access options in the case of hepaticojejunostomy or altered anatomy due to gastric bypass.[96,97]

SUMMARY

Refinements in surgical techniques, abandonment of routine use of T-tubes, advancements in postoperative care, and immunosuppression have led to a progressive decline in the incidence of overall complications after LT. However, biliary complications are still a common cause of morbidity and mortality in liver transplant recipients, frequently resulting in the need for multiple invasive interventions and in severe cases retransplantation. The discordance between organ availability and organ demand has increased the use of extended criteria donor grafts, living donor transplantation, and split LT, which pose additional risks for biliary complications. Endoscopic modalities are now the treatment of choice for biliary complications. The use of enteroscopy-assisted ERCP for choledocho-jejunal reconstruction in variant anatomy and the use of metal stents to treat refractory biliary are some of the newer approaches that have demonstrated consistent benefit and safety even in complex settings.

DISCLOSURE

The authors have nothing to disclose.

REFERENCES

1. Boeva I, Karagyozov PI, Tishkov I. Post-liver transplant biliary complications: current knowledge and therapeutic advances. World J Hepatol 2021;13(1):66–79.
2. Starzl TE, Iwatsuki S, Van Thiel DH, et al. Evolution of liver transplantation. Hepatology 1982;2(5):614–36.
3. Roos FJM, Poley JW, Polak WG, et al. Biliary complications after liver transplantation; recent developments in etiology, diagnosis and endoscopic treatment. Best Pract Res Clin Gastroenterol 2017;31(2):227–35.
4. Kwong AJ, Kim WR, Lake JR, et al. OPTN/SRTR 2019 annual data report: liver. Am J Transplant 2021;21(Suppl 2):208–315.
5. Jalan R, Gines P, Olson JC, et al. Acute-on chronic liver failure. J Hepatol 2012; 57(6):1336–48.
6. Pine JK, Aldouri A, Young AL, et al. Liver transplantation following donation after cardiac death: an analysis using matched pairs. Liver Transpl 2009;15(9):1072–82.
7. Starzl TE, Ishikawa M, Putnam CW, et al. Progress in and deterrents to orthotopic liver transplantation, with special reference to survival, resistance to hyperacute rejection, and biliary duct reconstruction. Transplant Proc 1974;6(4 Suppl 1): 129–39.
8. Jorgensen JE, Waljee AK, Volk ML, et al. Is MRCP equivalent to ERCP for diagnosing biliary obstruction in orthotopic liver transplant recipients? A meta-analysis. Gastrointest Endosc 2011;73(5):955–62.
9. Foley DP, Fernandez LA, Leverson G, et al. Biliary complications after liver transplantation from donation after cardiac death donors: an analysis of risk factors and long-term outcomes from a single center. Ann Surg 2011;253(4):817–25.
10. Abouljoud MS, Kim DY, Yoshida A, et al. Impact of aberrant arterial anatomy and location of anastomosis on technical outcomes after liver transplantation. J Gastrointest Surg 2005;9(5):672–8.
11. Verdonk RC, Buis CI, Porte RJ, et al. Anastomotic biliary strictures after liver transplantation: causes and consequences. Liver Transpl 2006;12(5):726–35.
12. Nakamura T, Iida T, Ushigome H, et al. Risk factors and management for biliary complications following adult living-donor liver transplantation. Ann Transplant 2017;22:671–6.
13. Park JS, Kim MH, Lee SK, et al. Efficacy of endoscopic and percutaneous treatments for biliary complications after cadaveric and living donor liver transplantation. Gastrointest Endosc 2003;57(1):78–85.
14. Verdonk RC, Buis CI, Porte RJ, et al. Biliary complications after liver transplantation: a review. Scand J Gastroenterol Suppl 2006;(243):89–101.

15. Pascher A, Neuhaus P. Biliary complications after deceased-donor orthotopic liver transplantation. J Hepatobiliary Pancreat Surg 2006;13(6):487–96.
16. Neuhaus P, Pascher A. Transplantation of the Liver. In: Transplantation of the Liver. 3 ed. Saunders; 2014:976-995.
17. Davidson BR, Rai R, Kurzawinski TR, et al. Prospective randomized trial of end-to-end versus side-to-side biliary reconstruction after orthotopic liver transplantation. Br J Surg 1999;86(4):447–52.
18. Shaked A. Use of T tube in liver transplantation. Liver Transpl Surg 1997;3(5 Suppl 1):S22–3.
19. Wells MM, Croome KP, Boyce E, et al. Roux-en-Y choledochojejunostomy versus duct-to-duct biliary anastomosis in liver transplantation for primary sclerosing cholangitis: a meta-analysis. Transplant Proc 2013;45(6):2263–71.
20. Ayoub WS, Esquivel CO, Martin P. Biliary complications following liver transplantation. Dig Dis Sci 2010;55(6):1540–6.
21. Guichelaar MM, Benson JT, Malinchoc M, et al. Risk factors for and clinical course of non-anastomotic biliary strictures after liver transplantation. Am J Transplant 2003;3(7):885–90.
22. Scatton O, Meunier B, Cherqui D, et al. Randomized trial of choledochocholedochostomy with or without a T tube in orthotopic liver transplantation. Ann Surg 2001;233(3):432–7.
23. Vougas V, Rela M, Gane E, et al. A prospective randomised trial of bile duct reconstruction at liver transplantation: T tube or no T tube? Transpl Int 1996; 9(4):392–5.
24. Qian YB, Liu CL, Lo CM, et al. Risk factors for biliary complications after liver transplantation. Arch Surg 2004;139(10):1101–5.
25. O'Connor TP, Lewis WD, Jenkins RL. Biliary tract complications after liver transplantation. Arch Surg 1995;130(3):312–7.
26. Amador A, Charco R, Marti J, et al. Cost/efficacy clinical trial about the use of T-tube in cadaveric donor liver transplant: preliminary results. Transplant Proc 2005;37(2):1129–30.
27. Porayko MK, Kondo M, Steers JL. Liver transplantation: late complications of the biliary tract and their management. Semin Liver Dis 1995;15(2):139–55.
28. Gámán G, Gelley F, Doros A, et al. Biliary complications after orthotopic liver transplantation: the Hungarian experience. Transplant Proc 2013;45(10):3695–7.
29. Singhal A, Stokes K, Sebastian A, et al. Endovascular treatment of hepatic artery thrombosis following liver transplantation. Transpl Int 2010;23(3):245–56.
30. Hejazi Kenari SK, Zimmerman A, Eslami M, et al. Current state of art management for vascular complications after liver transplantation. Middle East J Dig Dis 2014; 6(3):121–30.
31. Langnas AN, Marujo W, Stratta RJ, et al. Hepatic allograft rescue following arterial thrombosis. Role of urgent revascularization. Transplantation 1991;51(1):86–90.
32. Busuttil RW, Farmer DG, Yersiz H, et al. Analysis of long-term outcomes of 3200 liver transplantations over two decades: a single-center experience. Ann Surg 2005;241(6):905–16 [discussion: 916–8].
33. Saad WE, Saad NE, Davies MG, et al. Transhepatic balloon dilation of anastomotic biliary strictures in liver transplant recipients: the significance of a patent hepatic artery. J Vasc Interv Radiol 2005;16(9):1221–8.
34. Pareja E, Cortes M, Navarro R, et al. Vascular complications after orthotopic liver transplantation: hepatic artery thrombosis. Transplant Proc 2010;42(8):2970–2.

35. Duffy JP, Hong JC, Farmer DG, et al. Vascular complications of orthotopic liver transplantation: experience in more than 4,200 patients. J Am Coll Surg 2009; 208(5):896–903 [discussion: 903–5].

36. Panaro F, Gallix B, Bouyabrine H, et al. Liver transplantation and spontaneous neovascularization after arterial thrombosis: "the neovascularized liver. Transpl Int 2011;24(9):949–57.

37. Nüssler NC, Settmacher U, Haase R, et al. Diagnosis and treatment of arterial steal syndromes in liver transplant recipients. Liver Transpl 2003;9(6):596–602.

38. Aberg F, Mäkisalo H, Höckerstedt K, et al. Infectious complications more than 1 year after liver transplantation: a 3-decade nationwide experience. Am J Transplant 2011;11(2):287–95.

39. Bosch W, Heckman MG, Diehl NN, et al. Association of cytomegalovirus infection and disease with death and graft loss after liver transplant in high-risk recipients. Am J Transplant 2011;11(10):2181–9.

40. Gotthardt DN, Senft J, Sauer P, et al. Occult cytomegalovirus cholangitis as a potential cause of cholestatic complications after orthotopic liver transplantation? A study of cytomegalovirus DNA in bile. Liver Transpl 2013;19(10):1142–50.

41. Halme L, Hockerstedt K, Lautenschlager I. Cytomegalovirus infection and development of biliary complications after liver transplantation. Transplantation 2003; 75(11):1853–8.

42. O'Grady JG, Alexander GJ, Sutherland S, et al. Cytomegalovirus infection and donor/recipient HLA antigens: interdependent co-factors in pathogenesis of vanishing bile-duct syndrome after liver transplantation. Lancet 1988;2(8606):302–5.

43. Thuluvath PJ, Pfau PR, Kimmey MB, et al. Biliary complications after liver transplantation: the role of endoscopy. Endoscopy 2005;37(9):857–63.

44. Kochhar G, Parungao JM, Hanouneh IA, et al. Biliary complications following liver transplantation. World J Gastroenterol 2013;19(19):2841–6.

45. Potthoff A, Hahn A, Kubicka S, et al. Diagnostic value of ultrasound in detection of biliary tract complications after liver transplantation. Hepat Mon 2013;13(1): e6003.

46. Sharma S, Gurakar A, Jabbour N. Biliary strictures following liver transplantation: past, present and preventive strategies. Liver Transpl 2008;14(6):759–69.

47. Rerknimitr R, Sherman S, Fogel EL, et al. Biliary tract complications after orthotopic liver transplantation with choledochocholedochostomy anastomosis: endoscopic findings and results of therapy. Gastrointest Endosc 2002;55(2):224–31.

48. Boraschi P, Donati F, Gigoni R, et al. MR cholangiography in orthotopic liver transplantation: sensitivity and specificity in detecting biliary complications. Clin Transplant 2010;24(4):E82–7.

49. Seale MK, Catalano OA, Saini S, et al. Hepatobiliary-specific MR contrast agents: role in imaging the liver and biliary tree. Radiographics 2009;29(6):1725–48.

50. Sebagh M, Yilmaz F, Karam V, et al. The histologic pattern of "biliary tract pathology" is accurate for the diagnosis of biliary complications. Am J Surg Pathol 2005; 29(3):318–23.

51. Ostroff JW. Post-transplant biliary problems. Gastrointest Endosc Clin N Am 2001;11(1):163–83.

52. Williams EJ, Taylor S, Fairclough P, et al. Risk factors for complication following ERCP; results of a large-scale, prospective multicenter study. Endoscopy 2007; 39(9):793–801.

53. Freeman ML, Nelson DB, Sherman S, et al. Complications of endoscopic biliary sphincterotomy. N Engl J Med 1996;335(13):909–18.

54. Sanna C, Giordanino C, Giono I, et al. Safety and efficacy of endoscopic retrograde cholangiopancreatography in patients with post-liver transplant biliary complications: results of a cohort study with long-term follow-up. Gut Liver 2011;5(3):328–34.
55. Hüsing A, Cicinnati VR, Maschmeier M, et al. Complications after endoscopic sphincterotomy in liver transplant recipients: a retrospective single-centre study. Arab J Gastroenterol 2015;16(2):46–9.
56. Greif F, Bronsther OL, Van Thiel DH, et al. The incidence, timing, and management of biliary tract complications after orthotopic liver transplantation. Ann Surg 1994;219(1):40–5.
57. Ostroff JW, Roberts JP, Gordon RL, et al. The management of T tube leaks in orthotopic liver transplant recipients with endoscopically placed nasobiliary catheters. Transplantation 1990;49(5):922–4.
58. Banzo I, Blanco I, Gutiérrez-Mendiguchía C, et al. Hepatobiliary scintigraphy for the diagnosis of bile leaks produced after T-tube removal in orthotopic liver transplantation. Nucl Med Commun 1998;19(3):229–36.
59. Kanazawa A, Kubo S, Tanaka H, et al. Bile leakage after living donor liver transplantation demonstrated with hepatobiliary scan using 9mTc-PMT. Ann Nucl Med 2003;17(6):507–9.
60. Sendino O, Fernández-Simon A, Law R, et al. Endoscopic management of bile leaks after liver transplantation: an analysis of two high-volume transplant centers. United Eur Gastroenterol J 2018;6(1):89–96.
61. Akamatsu N, Sugawara Y, Hashimoto D. Biliary reconstruction, its complications and management of biliary complications after adult liver transplantation: a systematic review of the incidence, risk factors and outcome. Transpl Int 2011;24(4):379–92.
62. Krok KL, Cárdenas A, Thuluvath PJ. Endoscopic management of biliary complications after liver transplantation. Clin Liver Dis 2010;14(2):359–71.
63. Luigiano C, Bassi M, Ferrara F, et al. Placement of a new fully covered self-expanding metal stent for postoperative biliary strictures and leaks not responding to plastic stenting. Surg Laparosc Endosc Percutan Tech 2013;23(2):159–62.
64. Saab S, Martin P, Soliman GY, et al. Endoscopic management of biliary leaks after T-tube removal in liver transplant recipients: nasobiliary drainage versus biliary stenting. Liver Transpl 2000;6(5):627–32.
65. Morelli J, Mulcahy HE, Willner IR, et al. Endoscopic treatment of post-liver transplantation biliary leaks with stent placement across the leak site. Gastrointest Endosc 2001;54(4):471–5.
66. Copelan A, Bahoura L, Tardy F, et al. Etiology, diagnosis, and management of bilomas: a current update. Tech Vasc Interv Radiol 2015;18(4):236–43.
67. Londoño MC, Balderramo D, Cárdenas A. Management of biliary complications after orthotopic liver transplantation: the role of endoscopy. World J Gastroenterol 2008;14(4):493–7.
68. Chen XP, Peng SY, Peng CH, et al. A ten-year study on non-surgical treatment of postoperative bile leakage. World J Gastroenterol 2002;8(5):937–42.
69. Simoes P, Kesar V, Ahmad J. Spectrum of biliary complications following live donor liver transplantation. World J Hepatol 2015;7(14):1856–65.
70. Jagannath S, Kalloo AN. Biliary complications after liver transplantation. Curr Treat Options Gastroenterol 2002;5(2):101–12.
71. Bourgeois N, Deviére J, Yeaton P, et al. Diagnostic and therapeutic endoscopic retrograde cholangiography after liver transplantation. Gastrointest Endosc 1995;42(6):527–34.

72. Schwartz DA, Petersen BT, Poterucha JJ, et al. Endoscopic therapy of anastomotic bile duct strictures occurring after liver transplantation. Gastrointest Endosc 2000;51(2):169–74.

73. Bortolasi L, Violi P, Carraro A, et al. Complications and outcomes of endoscopic treatment in a cohort of patients with biliary stenosis after orthotopic liver transplant: a retrospective observational study. Exp Clin Transplant 2019;17(4): 513–21.

74. Alazmi WM, Fogel EL, Watkins JL, et al. Recurrence rate of anastomotic biliary strictures in patients who have had previous successful endoscopic therapy for anastomotic narrowing after orthotopic liver transplantation. Endoscopy 2006; 38(6):571–4.

75. Pascher A, Neuhaus P. Bile duct complications after liver transplantation. Transpl Int 2005;18(6):627–42.

76. Rizk RS, McVicar JP, Emond MJ, et al. Endoscopic management of biliary strictures in liver transplant recipients: effect on patient and graft survival. Gastrointest Endosc 1998;47(2):128–35.

77. Pfau PR, Kochman ML, Lewis JD, et al. Endoscopic management of postoperative biliary complications in orthotopic liver transplantation. Gastrointest Endosc 2000;52(1):55–63.

78. Graziadei IW, Schwaighofer H, Koch R, et al. Long-term outcome of endoscopic treatment of biliary strictures after liver transplantation. Liver Transpl 2006;12(5): 718–25.

79. Cotton PB, Elta GH, Carter CR, et al. Rome IV. Gallbladder and sphincter of Oddi disorders. Gastroenterology 2016. https://doi.org/10.1053/j.gastro.2016.02.033.

80. Bozkurt T, Orth KH, Butsch B, et al. Long-term clinical outcome of postcholecystectomy patients with biliary-type pain: results of manometry, noninvasive techniques and endoscopic sphincterotomy. Eur J Gastroenterol Hepatol 1996;8(3):245–9.

81. Sheng R, Ramirez CB, Zajko AB, et al. Biliary stones and sludge in liver transplant patients: a 13-year experience. Radiology 1996;198(1):243–7.

82. Yang YL, Shi LJ, Lin MJ, et al. Clinical analysis and significance of cholangiography for biliary cast/stone after orthotopic liver transplantation. J Nanosci Nanotechnol 2013;13(1):171–7.

83. Cao S, Cox K, So SS, et al. Potential effect of cyclosporin A in formation of cholesterol gallstones in pediatric liver transplant recipients. Dig Dis Sci 1997;42(7): 1409–15.

84. Doyle MB, Maynard E, Lin Y, et al. Outcomes with split liver transplantation are equivalent to those with whole organ transplantation. J Am Coll Surg 2013; 217(1):102–12 [discussion: 113–4].

85. Shah SA, Levy GA, Adcock LD, et al. Adult-to-adult living donor liver transplantation. Can J Gastroenterol 2006;20(5):339–43.

86. Freise CE, Gillespie BW, Koffron AJ, et al. Recipient morbidity after living and deceased donor liver transplantation: findings from the A2ALL Retrospective Cohort Study. Am J Transplant 2008;8(12):2569–79.

87. Aparício DPDS, Otoch JP, Montero EFS, et al. Endoscopic approach for management of biliary strictures in liver transplant recipients: a systematic review and meta-analysis. United Eur Gastroenterol J 2017;5(6):827–45.

88. Tashiro H, Itamoto T, Sasaki T, et al. Biliary complications after duct-to-duct biliary reconstruction in living-donor liver transplantation: causes and treatment. World J Surg 2007;31(11):2222–9.

89. Wadhawan M, Kumar A, Gupta S, et al. Post-transplant biliary complications: an analysis from a predominantly living donor liver transplant center. J Gastroenterol Hepatol 2013;28(6):1056–60.

90. Yazumi S, Yoshimoto T, Hisatsune H, et al. Endoscopic treatment of biliary complications after right-lobe living-donor liver transplantation with duct-to-duct biliary anastomosis. J Hepatobiliary Pancreat Surg 2006;13(6):502–10.

91. Tsujino T, Isayama H, Kogure H, et al. Endoscopic management of biliary strictures after living donor liver transplantation. Clin J Gastroenterol 2017;10(4): 297–311.

92. Hüsing-Kabar A, Heinzow HS, Schmidt HH, et al. Single-operator cholangioscopy for biliary complications in liver transplant recipients. World J Gastroenterol 2017;23(22):4064–71.

93. Aljebreen AM, Alharbi OR, Azzam N, et al. Efficacy of spyglass-guided electrohydraulic lithotripsy in difficult bile duct stones. Saudi J Gastroenterol 2014;20(6): 366–70.

94. Saleem A, Baron TH, Gostout CJ, et al. Endoscopic retrograde cholangiopancreatography using a single-balloon enteroscope in patients with altered Roux-en-Y anatomy. Endoscopy 2010;42(8):656–60.

95. Hüsing A, Cicinnati VR, Beckebaum S, et al. Endoscopic ultrasound: valuable tool for diagnosis of biliary complications in liver transplant recipients? Surg Endosc 2015;29(6):1433–8.

96. Attam R, Leslie D, Freeman M, et al. EUS-assisted, fluoroscopically guided gastrostomy tube placement in patients with Roux-en-Y gastric bypass: a novel technique for access to the gastric remnant. Gastrointest Endosc 2011;74(3):677–82.

97. Sondhi AR, Sonnenday CJ, Parikh ND, et al. EUS-guided gastrojejunal anastomosis to facilitate endoscopic retrograde cholangiography in a patient with a right lobe liver transplant and Roux-en-Y anatomy. VideoGIE 2020;5(10):473–5.

Endoscopic Ultrasound-Guided Biliary Interventions in Liver Disease

Shyam Vedantam, DO[a], Sunil Amin, MD, MPH[b],*

KEYWORDS

- Endoscopic ultrasound • EUS • ERCP
- Endoscopic retrograde cholangiopancreatography • Choledocoduodenostomy
- Hepaticogastrostomy • EUS-guided gallbladder drainage • Therapeutic endoscopy

KEY POINTS

- Endoscopic retrograde cholangiopancreatography (ERCP) is the current first choice for patients with jaundice caused by biliary obstruction, but it may be unsuccessful due to a variety of reasons.
- The current second choice for relieving biliary obstruction is percutaneous drainage, which has its own drawbacks.
- Endoscopic ultrasonography-guided biliary drainage (EUS-BD) (choledocoduodenostomy or hepaticogastrostomy) is emerging as an alternative option to percutaneous drainage with studies showing similar technical and clinical success between the 2 options.
- In patients with acute cholecystitis who are not surgical candidates and who would otherwise be managed with percutaneous cholecystostomy, EUS-guided transmural gallbladder drainage is an emerging modality that may offer better clinical success with lower rates of recurrent cholecystitis.
- In expert centers and/or those with trained advanced endoscopists, EUS-BD can be attempted as a second-line option for biliary decompression.

INTRODUCTION

Biliary obstruction can be caused by pancreatic, biliary tract, or gallbladder (GB) malignancies, along with other benign causes (both intra- and extrahepatic). Endoscopic retrograde cholangiopancreatography (ERCP) is the first-line procedure to alleviate the biliary obstruction. Technical success, defined as bile duct cannulation, is greater than 90%, whereas periprocedural and postprocedural complication rates are approximately 2% and 10%, respectively.[1] The reported rate of ERCP-induced

a Department of Medicine, University of Miami, Miami, FL, USA; b Division of Digestive Health and Liver Diseases, Department of Medicine, University of Miami, 1120 NW 14th Street, Clinical Research Building, Suite 11145 (D-49), Miami, FL 33136, USA
* Corresponding author.
E-mail address: sunil.amin@med.miami.edu

Clin Liver Dis 26 (2022) 101–114
https://doi.org/10.1016/j.cld.2021.08.009
1089-3261/22/© 2021 Elsevier Inc. All rights reserved.

pancreatitis is approximately 4.5% (which confers a 4.4% mortality rate of that subset).[2] However, increased difficulty of the ERCP increases the rate of complications. For example, studies have shown that the aforementioned pancreatitis rate in ERCP is achieved when the selective biliary cannulation is achieved in less than 5 minutes, but increases to greater than 10% if the procedure takes more than 10 minutes or requires more than 10 attempts at biliary cannulation.[3,4] ERCP can fail in a variety of instances—surgically altered anatomy, duodenal obstruction, inaccessible papilla due to malignancy, or cannulation failure to name a few.[5] Even when ERCP is technically successful with the placement of a stent, recurrent obstruction can occur in up to 41% based on a Cochrane review—a significant burden on already frail patients and a considerable morbidity factor.[6]

The decision for the next step after the failure of ERCP is largely based on individual preference, level of training, and expertise. Other ERCP-based biliary access techniques that can be conducted during the initial procedure include pancreatic guidewire assisted cannulation (double-wire technique), transpancreatic septotomy, and needle-knife fistulotomy or precut papillotomy.[7] In a meta-analysis studying these techniques, transpancreatic sphincterotomy demonstrated higher biliary cannulation rate, but a similar safety profile in the short term among all these advanced ERCP-based biliary access techniques (no long-term data were available for analysis).[8] In patients who had a failed ERCP, other than reattempting ERCP, the current practice model is to turn to percutaneous transhepatic biliary drainage (PTBD) by interventional radiology.[9]

Similarly, although laparoscopic cholecystectomy (LC) is the standard treatment for acute cholecystitis, a significant portion of these patients are not surgical candidates due to the significant morbidity and mortality in those who are high risk.[10] One option is intravenous fluids and antibiotics to delay LC until the patient has recovered and is prepared for surgery.[11] However, GB drainage must be added for those who do not improve after a few days of nonoperative management due to the risk of further deterioration and sepsis.[12,13] Patients with chronic liver disease, particularly those with decompensated cirrhosis, pose an important challenge to the management of acute cholecystitis, as they are typically at high risk for surgical complications. In these patients, percutaneous cholecystectomy (PC) drains have been the most widely used intervention; however, endoscopic ultrasonography-guided GB drainage (EUS-GB) is emerging as a new modality that offers similar rates of technical and clinical success as PC with less need for recurrent intervention and increased patient satisfaction.[14–16]

THERAPEUTIC OPTIONS IN ENDOSCOPIC ULTRASOUND-GUIDED BILIARY ACCESS

The first description of EUS-guided biliary access is from 2001 by Giovannini and colleagues, but the procedures have gained more prominence within the past decade[17] This includes EUS-guided rendezvous (EUS-RV), EUS-guided anterograde stent/intervention (EUS-AG), EUS-guided choledocoduodenostomy (EUS-CDS), and EUS-guided hepaticogastrostomy (EUS-HG). Endoscopic ultrasonography-guided biliary drainage (EUS-BD) can be thought of in 2 categories: intra and extrahepatic (**Table 1**). In the intrahepatic approach, the left lobe of the liver is accessed through the gastric wall (or, uncommonly, through distal esophagus or jejunum). Examples of this are EUS-HG and EUS-AG. In the extrahepatic approach, the common bile duct is accessed through the duodenum. Examples of this are EUS-CDS and EUS-RV.

These procedures offer the advantage of being able to be performed during the index procedure after ERCP failure rather than needing to be scheduled at a future date. By bypassing the tumor site, they may avoid delayed stent dysfunction from tumor

Table 1		
Classification of different methods of EUS-guided biliary interventions		
An Overview of EUS-Guided Biliary Interventions		
EUS-Guided Biliary Drainage		
Intrahepatic Approach	The left lobe of the liver is accessed through the gastric wall, distal esophagus, or jejunum	• EUS-HG • EUS-AG
Extrahepatic Approach	The common bile duct is accessed through the duodenum	• EUS-CDS • EUS-RGV
EUS-Guided Gallbladder Drainage		
Extrahepatic Approach	The gallbladder is accessed transmurally through the stomach or duodenum	• EUS-GB

Abbreviations: EUS-HG, EUS-guided hepaticogastrostomy; EUS-AG, EUS-guided anterograde stent/ intervention; EUS-CDS, EUS-guided choledocoduodenostomy; EUS-RGV, EUS-guided rendezvous; EUS-GB, EUS-guided transmural gallbladder drainage.

tissue ingrowth.[18] The focus of this review will be on EUS-CDS and EUS-HG as these are the more well-researched EUS-guided biliary obstruction relief procedures.

Endoscopic Ultrasonography-Guided Rendezvous

EUS-RV can only be performed if the papilla can be accessed. The bile duct is punctured under EUS-guidance usually with a 19 gauge needle.[7] Contrast is injected to obtain a cholangiogram. A guidewire is then advanced through the papilla while leaving an excess tail to ensure stability while exchanging echoendoscope for duodenoscope. Access into the biliary system is then obtained by cannulating alongside this guidewire or grasping the tail through the duodenoscope channel for over-the-wire cannulation. EUS-RV may fail due to the inability to negotiate the guidewire across the stricture or papilla.

Endoscopic Ultrasonography-Guided Antegrade Drainage

EUS-AG drainage involves making a puncture tract into the intrahepatic bile duct, guide-wire advancement across the stricture/papilla, and possible over-the-wire dilation.[7] Whatever ERCP intervention (eg, stricture sampling or dilation) was previously attempted and failed is now performed over this new tract. This technique seems to have a lower success rate than the other EUS-guided techniques.[19]

Endoscopic Ultrasonography-Guided Choledocoduodenostomy and EUS-Guided Hepaticogastrostomy

Both EUS-CDS and EUS-HG are methods of transluminal biliary drainage (**Fig. 1**). Both place a stent across a puncture route to create a new drainage tract between the biliary and gastrointestinal tracts.[7] A puncture site is made with EUS guidance. A guidewire is then advanced through this tract so that a catheter, balloon, or cautery device can be advanced to dilate the puncture tract. A stent is then placed to create this new route of biliary drainage.

Endoscopic Ultrasonography-Guided Transmural Gallbladder Drainage

Alternatives to LC include PC, ERCP with transpapillary drainage (ETP), and EUS-guided transmural gallbladder drainage (EUS-GB). During EUS-GB, a puncture site is made through the stomach or duodenal walls, avoiding visible vessels, into the GB.[11] A guidewire is then passed through and coiled in the GB fundus so that the tract

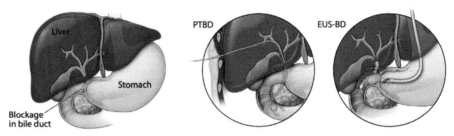

Fig. 1. EUS-CDS and EUS-HG. (*From* Wang K, Zhu J, Xing L, Wang Y, Jin Z, Li Z. Assessment of efficacy and safety of EUS-guided biliary drainage: A systematic review. *Gastrointest Endosc.* 2016;83(6):12181227. https://doi.org/10.1016/j.gie.2015.10.033.)

may be dilated and eventually stented with a lumen-apposing metal stent (LAMS) (**Fig. 2**).

CLINICAL OUTCOMES
Improvement with Experience—a Learning Curve

As previously mentioned, the first descriptions of these procedures began after 2001.[17] A multi-center survey study showed that endoscopists who had performed less than 20 EUS-BD procedures had a technical success of 67%, clinical success of 63%, and complications in 23% of patients.[20] It was reported in the study that the most common cause of technical failure was unsuccessful manipulation of the guidewire and that most complications were due to the transmural fistula.

Another single-center study also described the learning curve present in performing EUS-BD. Over a 5-year time span, 2 endoscopists retrospectively analyzed success and complication rates. In the first 3 years of the study, the failure and complication rates were 38% and 54%, respectively; this decreased to 11% and 22%, respectively, in the last 2 years.[21] These data imply that more experience results in more favorable outcomes. Furthermore, one meta-analysis of the efficacy and safety of EUS-BD

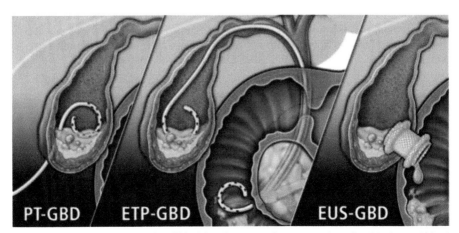

Fig. 2. EUS-guided transmural gallbladder drainage. (*From* Han SY, Kim SO, So H, Shin E, Kim DU, Park DH. EUS-guided biliary drainage versus ERCP for first-line palliation of malignant distal biliary obstruction: A systematic review and meta-analysis. *Sci Rep.* 2019;9(1):1-9. https://doi.org/10.1038/s41598-019-52993-x.)

analyzed the differences between studies before and after 2013.[22] It was seen that while the functional success and adverse event rates were not statistically significantly different, the technical success rate was higher in studies after 2013 (96.14% vs 90.68%).

Indeed, a single-center experience published this year reported a technical success rate of 97% and a complication rate of 12.9%.[22] All in all, this may point to EUS-BD becoming more efficacious and safe as training and patient selection, procedure organization, and EUS-BD tools improve.

Technical and Clinical Success of Endoscopic Ultrasonography-Guided Biliary Drainage

As discussed earlier, ERCP is the reference procedure with technical success, perioperative complication, and postoperative complication rates of approximately 90%, 2%, and 10%, respectively.[1] A 2019 meta-analysis identified 17 studies for a total of 686 patients who underwent EUS-BD.[23] The analysis reported technical and clinical success rates for EUS-HG as 96% (95% confidence interval (CI): 93–98) and 84% (95% CI: 80–88), respectively. The technical and clinical success rates for EUS-CDS were reported as 95% (95% CI: 91–97) and 87% (95% CI: 82–91), respectively. Of note, reported adverse event rates were significantly higher ($P = .01$) for EUS-HG (29%, 95% CI: 24–34) than EUS-CDS (20%, 95% CI: 16–25). It was noted that most of the adverse events in EUS-HG were due to stent dysfunction, which may have been due to stent choice rather than the EUS-BD technique.

Endoscopic Ultrasonography-Guided Biliary Drainage Versus Percutaneous Transhepatic Biliary Drainage in Biliary Obstruction

If ERCP fails, there is no consensus on the optimal salvage intervention: EUS-BD versus PTBD. PTBD has reported technical, clinical, and adverse event rates of 96%, 95.7%, and 18.3%, respectively.[24] A 2017 meta-analysis analyzed 9 studies for a total of 483 patients to examine this clinical question.[25] There was no difference in technical success between the 2 procedures (odds ratio (OR): 1.78, 95% CI: 0.69–4.59). However, EUS-BD was associated with better clinical success (OR: 0.45, 95% CI: 0.23–0.89), fewer postprocedure adverse events (OR: 0.23, 95% CI: 0.12–0.47), and lower rates of reintervention (OR: 0.13, 95% CI: 0.07–0.24). No difference was noted in hospital length of stay; however, EUS-BD was more cost-effective than PTBD with a pooled standard mean difference of −0.63 (95% CI: 1.06–0.2). The increase in cost associated with PTBD is driven by the need for more reinterventions such as catheter changes. There were distinct differences among the studies though. Two were multicenter studies, whereas the other 7 were single-center based. Different methods and procedures of EUS-BD were used in the included studies: both intra and extrahepatic approaches were used, different types of stent usages in the PTBD group versus metal stents exclusively in the EUS-BD group, and inclusion of benign and/or malignant etiologies in some.

Sharaiha and colleagues explain the secondary benefits of the above findings. As EUS-BD is associated with a lower rate of reinterventions and a better rate of clinical success, this would to timelier biliary drainage, which is especially helpful in malignancy cases whereby chemotherapy can be initiated earlier and with stronger regimens. For example, in locally advanced pancreatic cancer, FOLFIRINOX is one of the most effective regimens, but the irinotecan component should be withheld if the serum bilirubin is greater than 1.5 times the upper limit of normal.[26] Optimal biliary drainage, and its delays due to stent dysfunction, may be an increasingly limiting step in starting neoadjuvant therapy and oncologic outcomes.[18] This longitudinal benefit does not appear to have been studied as of yet, but is a future direction of the study of EUS-BD.

An additional benefit with EUS than PTBD is the quality of life. There are frequently minor problems with PTBD that require a premature exchange of drains in almost half of cases, which can affect patients' quality of life.[27] PTBD also requires an external drain (and subsequent bag exchanges) than the internal drain of EUS-BD.

Primary Endoscopic Retrograde Cholangiopancreatography Versus Endoscopic Ultrasonography-Guided Biliary Drainage

ERCP is the first-line modality for biliary access and decompression, but EUS-BD is emerging as a modality for salvage therapy. Interestingly, a recent meta-analysis sought to evaluate if EUS-BD could be used as the primary option for biliary decompression.[28,29] Both primary ERCP and EUS-BD achieved similar levels of technical success (96.5% vs 94.8%, respectively), clinical success (95.7% vs 93.8%, respectively), and adverse outcomes (18.3% vs 16.3%, respectively), as well as similar odds of requiring reintervention for biliary drainage (OR: 1.68 with 95% CI: 0.76–3.73). Despite these similarities, there were some notable differences: 9.5% of patients developed procedure-related pancreatitis in the ERCP group versus 0% in the EUS-BD group; there was no significant difference in the nonpancreatitis-related adverse events. This observation is explained by the fact that EUS-BD does not involve any manipulation of the ampulla/pancreatic orifice. Kakked and colleagues demonstrated that while the pooled reintervention rates between the EUS-BD and ERCP groups (15.6% vs 22.6%, respectively) did not achieve statistical significance, the causes for reinterventions were different.[28] The ERCP group had significantly higher odds of requiring reintervention due to tumor overgrowth (OR: 5.35, 95% CI: 1.64–17.50). On the other hand, the ERCP group had significantly lower odds of requiring reintervention due to stent migration than the EUS-BD group (OR: 0.16, 95% CI: 0.04–0.76). The incidences of acute cholangitis, cholecystitis, biloma, and bleeding were too low for meaningful comparison between the groups. Of note, all studies in the ERCP group used self-expanding metal stents (SEMS), which included a mixture of covered, uncovered, and partially covered SEMS. Other benefits were also noted in that study. Those in the ERCP group were less likely to receive systemic chemotherapy than the EUS-BD group (OR: 0.57, 95% CI: 0.34–0.95).[28] Although admittedly a small study of 125 patients, quality of life was better in the group that underwent EUS-BD than ERCP 12 weeks after the procedure.[30]

A different meta-analysis went on to investigate stent-related outcomes in primary EUS-BD versus ERCP. Miller and colleagues reported EUS-BD was associated with decreased stent/catheter dysfunction requiring reintervention (relative risk (RR): 0.41, 95% CI: 0.23–0.74) or tumor in-growth (RR: 0.18, 95% CI: 0.06–0.62).[18] This may offer a morbidity benefit in frail patients.

Endoscopic Ultrasonography-Guided Transmural Gallbladder Drainage Versus Percutaneous Cholecystectomy Versus Laparoscopic Cholecystectomy in Acute Cholecystitis

Nonoperative methods for GB drainage have been investigated for over a decade.[31] Patients with decompensated liver disease are among other groups that are at high risk for surgical complications and typically require nonoperative interventions for the treatment of acute cholecystitis. A recent network meta-analysis by Podboy and colleagues attempted to clarify the differences between PC, ETP, and EUS-GB for acute cholecystitis.[32] Ten studies were included for a total of 1267 patients. PC and

EUS-GB had higher likelihoods of technical and clinical success than ETP (EUS-GB vs PC vs ETP: 2.00 vs 1.02 vs 2.89). Technical success was defined as the ability to access and drain the GB with immediate drainage of bile; clinical success was defined as a resolution of clinical symptoms and/or improvement in biochemical parameters. EUS-GB had the lowest risk of recurrent cholecystitis (EUS-GB vs PC vs ETP: 1.09 vs 2.02 vs 2.89). Furthermore, PC had the highest risk of reintervention (EUS-GB vs PC vs ETP: 1.81 vs 2.99 vs 2.89) and unplanned readmissions (EUS-GB vs PC vs ETP: 1.58 vs 2.94 vs 1.47). ETP had the lowest mortality rate (EUS-GB vs PC vs ETP: 2.62 vs 2.09 vs 1.29). Overall, EUS-GB was associated with higher rates of clinical success and lower rates of recurrent episodes of cholecystitis. The authors suggested that while different clinical scenarios might influence one method over another, EUS-GB may be preferred in patients who are not planned to ultimately undergo cholecystectomy because of significant comorbidities (over PC) as the rates of recurrent cholecystitis, reinterventions, and unplanned admissions were lower.

A second study compared EUS-GB to LC using a propensity score matching analysis.[33] Technical and clinical success rates, lengths of hospital stay, 30-day adverse events, and mortality rates were similar between the 2 groups. There were also no differences in recurrent biliary events, reinterventions, and unplanned admissions in 1 year. Another benefit of EUS-GB is that the GB could be cleared of the remaining gallstones by cholecystoscopy through the stent during a subsequent procedure.[34] Although small, this study suggests that EUS-GB could be a viable alternative to LC for patients who are poor surgical candidates.

TECHNICAL CONSIDERATIONS
Anticoagulation

There are several guidelines for antithrombotic management in endoscopy, including the Japan Gastroenterological Endoscopy Society guidelines that classify EUS-BD as high-risk procedures.[35,36] A recent study of 220 patients (18 on anticoagulation) evaluated bleeding outcomes in patients undergoing EUS-BD.[37] Only one patient (5.5%) in the antithrombotic group and 2 (0.9%) in the nonantithrombotic group experienced moderate bleeding events, which was not statistically significant. This unchanged bleeding risk profile was also shown in separate case series that investigated the bleeding risk of EUS-GB in acute cholecystitis.[38,39]

Stent Options

Different types of stents have been used for decades in ERCP and other gastrointestinal procedures. There are inherent differences that may lead to the preference of one type of stent over the other. SEMS are preferred over plastic stents for EUS-BD as the wider lumen of SEMS reduces the risk of stent obstruction and the silicone covering reduces the risk of bile leak.[40] However, traditional SEMS lack flanges at their ends and migration is a major concern. On this note, a meta-analysis showed that stent migration and sludge formation are more common in covered versus uncovered SEMS (OR: 5.11, 95% CI: 1.84–14.17; OR: 2.46, 95% CI: 1.37–4.43).[41] The same study showed that covered SEMS have a higher rate of tumor overgrowth (OR: 2.00, 95% CI: 1.15–3.48), but a lower rate of tumor ingrowth (OR: 0.21, 95% CI: 0.09–0.50) compared with uncovered SEMS. Ultimately though, the rates of procedure-related adverse events were similar between groups.

LAMS are fully covered, dumbbell-shaped stents with perpendicular flanges, designed to mitigate the risk of migration.[42] Anderloni and colleagues describe a two-step process with the puncture of the bile duct and stent placement.[43]

Krishnamoorthi *and colleagues* performed a meta-analysis on LAMS in EUS-CDS.[40] Seven studies on EUS-CDS for a total of 284 patients were included. Pooled technical success, clinical success, and adverse event rates were 95.7% (95% CI: 93.2–98.1), 95.9% (95% CI: 92.8–98.9), and 5.2% (95% CI: 2.6–7.9), respectively. The authors caution the success of this technique though in those without significant biliary dilation as misdeployment can result in bile leak or duodenal perforation. There have been reports of bleeding in LAMS in draining pancreatic fluid collections.[44] This was not replicated in the Krishnamoorthi *and colleagues* meta-analysis. This is postulated to be due to the difference in vessel locations and the incidence of pseudoaneurysms in pancreatic fluid collections.[40]

Smaller studies have sought to identify if other stent variations could improve outcomes. Recently, one study assessed the addition of a double-pigtail stent within a LAMS for the palliative management of biliary obstruction.[45] However, there was no difference in clinical success, adverse event, recurrent biliary obstruction, or survival rate. Therefore, this technical variant does not seem to offer any therapeutic benefit. Another small study used a novel double-bare, covered SEMS (DBSEMS) and found that in 22 patients who underwent EUS-CDS, DBSEMS may prevent cholangitis due to stent kinking and increased stent patency than fully covered stents.[46]

Limitations of Endoscopic Ultrasonography-Guided Biliary Drainage

EUS-BD is a technically difficult procedure. An editorial summed up several obstacles in making EUS-BD a widely-performed technique.[47] First, the acuteness of the angle between the aspiration needle and the bile duct can result in accidental shearing of the guidewire. Second, the transduodenal approach can make the rendezvous passage of the guidewire through the major papilla technically difficult (as the guidewire preferentially goes into the intrahepatic bile ducts because of the direction of the needle). The creation of a transmural fistula with a graded-dilation approach can be difficult, and the alternative use of electrocautery carries its own inherent risks. Additionally, overly aggressive dilation can result in bile leak or perforation. The deployment of a stent may occlude the cystic duct stump in those patients with a distended GB, causing stent-induced cholecystitis.

There are limited devices to perform the technique. Moreover, not all products are available at all institutions. Stents of different sizes may be more appropriate for dilated or nondilated bile ducts, but the optimal size may not be available. As such, there is no standardized approach to the technical aspects of the procedure. With the advent of new devices, there may be a more uniform, technically feasible procedure to follow. For example, in a study of 32 patients, the procedural time was significantly shorter (10 vs 15 minutes), and there was no difference in the technical success, clinical success, or adverse event rates, for those who underwent EUS-BD with the new device versus conventional 8.5 French biliary stent introducer with a fully covered metal stent. This device has a tapered metal tip that functions as a push-type dilator without the need for dilation, use of electrocautery, or fistula tract dilation after needle puncture; the preloaded SEMS has an uncovered portion to allow for better anchoring and to prevent occlusion of side branches in the biliary tree; and the covered portion extends transmurally to prevent intraperitoneal leakage of bile.[30,48] Paik and colleagues demonstrated the use of one-step dedicated stent introducer (DEUS; Standard Sci Tech Inc., Seoul, South Korea) in a randomized-controlled clinical trial and showed that their EUS-BD technique had improved outcomes (lower rates of postprocedure pancreatitis and reintervention, as well as higher rate of stent patency) than ERCP.[30]

DISCUSSION

ERCP will likely remain the gold standard for biliary decompression (**Fig. 3**). However, as the rate of duodenal stenosis in pancreatic malignancies is 13% to 20%, it may behoove endoscopists to pursue primary EUS-BD (or at least consider the necessity) in these patients as ERCP may not be possible.[49] If the ultimate goal is surgical resection in pancreatic malignancies, EUS-CDS may be preferred over ERCP as the former has a lower rate of precipitating pancreatitis (a major cause of delay during the preoperative period) and has been shown to not interfere with subsequent pancreaticoduodenectomy.[29,50] A summary of the technical, clinical, and adverse event rates of the different procedures mentioned above is included in **Table 2**.

Choosing the route of access for EUS-BD will depend on a variety of factors. First (and likely most importantly), it will depend on the individual endoscopist's training, expertise, and comfort level with each procedure. Second, it will depend on the resources available at that center—equipment necessary for each procedure, equipment that might optimize one technique versus another, and backup specialists (interventional radiologists, advanced gastrointestinal surgeons). Patients with hilar biliary obstruction, history of gastric bypass, and gastric outlet obstruction are increasingly being treated with EUS-HG. If the biliary obstruction appears to be more distally located, then at least one meta-analysis favors EUS-CDS due to potentially lower adverse event rate.[51] Furthermore, the EUS-CDS technique may be easier technically due to the smaller excursion between the duodenum and bile duct in comparison to the excursion between the stomach and the liver.[40] Additionally, the increased adoption of a one-step device and innovation in the device industry may make certain techniques more feasible.

Different anatomical-based algorithms have been proposed.[52,53] Tyberg and colleagues have proposed an algorithm based on the imaging of anatomic findings to help guide and standardize the method of EUS-BD after ERCP failure (**Fig. 4**).[52] The first step is to obtain cross-sectional imaging. The authors suggest an extrahepatic

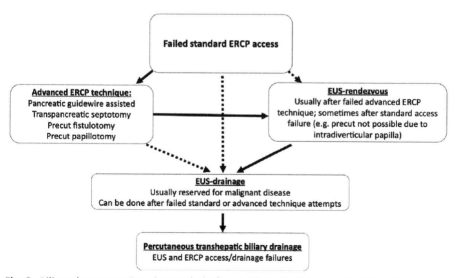

Fig. 3. Biliary decompression. (*From* El Chafic AH, Shah JN. Advances in Biliary Access. *Curr Gastroenterol Rep.* 2020;22(12). https://doi.org/10.1007/s11894-020-00800-3.)

Table 2
Reported technical, clinical, and adverse event rates for each technique

	ERCP[25]	PTBD[21]	EUS-CDS[20]	EUS-HG[20]	PC[28]	EUS-GB
Technical Success Rate	97%	95%	95%	96%	98%	95%
Clinical Success Rate	96%	95%	87%	84%	89%	97%
Adverse Event Rate	18%	10%–31%	20%	29%	15%	12%

Abbreviations: ERCP, endoscopic retrograde cholangiopancreatography; EUS-CDS, EUS-guided choledocoduodenostomy; EUS-GB, EUS-guided transmural gallbladder drainage; EUS-HG, EUS-guided hepaticogastrostomy; PC, percutaneous cholecystectomy; PTBD, percutaneous transhepatic biliary drainage.

approach (EUS-CDS or EUS-RV) if imaging shows a nondilated intrahepatic biliary tree. If imaging shows a dilated intrahepatic duct, then antegrade placement of stent should be attempted. If this fails, EUS-HG should then be attempted. If this also fails, then either EUS-RV or EUS-CDS can be attempted. This algorithm has not been validated by any additional studies yet. However, as the meta-analysis by Hedjoude and colleagues notes, EUS-HG may have a higher adverse event rate.[23] Therefore, if anatomy allows, EUS-CDS may be optimal. However, if there is hilar biliary or duodenal obstruction, then endoscopists may consider EUS-HG over repeat ERCP or PTBD.

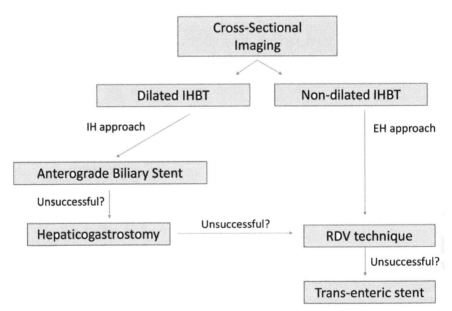

Fig. 4. EUS-BD after ERCP failure. EH, extra-hepatic; IH, intra-hepatic; IHBT, intra-hepatic biliary tree; RDV, rendez-vous. (*From* Bang JY, Navaneethan U, Hasan M, Hawes R, Varadarajulu S. Stent placement by EUS or ERCP for primary biliary decompression in pancreatic cancer: a randomized trial (with videos). *Gastrointest Endosc.* 2018;88(1):9-17. https://doi.org/10.1016/j.gie.2018.03.012.)

FUTURE DIRECTIONS

Advanced endoscopy is an evolving field. EUS-BD is on the frontier of becoming more popular and increasingly used as more endoscopists gain experience in the technique. With the evidence noted here, EUS-BD should be considered in the management of specific cases of biliary obstruction. Unless there is a contraindication to endoscopy such as frailty or limited survival benefit, EUS-BD can be used. Future research efforts should attempt to use new (easier to use) stent deployment devices to demonstrate that these techniques can be brought from select tertiary academic centers to the rest of the endoscopy community. Future studies can also take a holistic, longitudinal, and multidisciplinary approach to see if EUS-BD may improve surgical and morbidity outcomes.

CLINICS CARE POINTS

- ERCP will likely remain the overall first tool in biliary decompression due to the technical difficulty of and lack of dedicated instrumentation for EUS-BD procedures.
- EUS-BD is an emerging therapeutic option with similar rates of technical success, clinical success, and adverse event rates compared to ERCP and PTBD in expert hands. Therefore, based on the individual endoscopist's training and institutional resources, EUS-BD should be considered for biliary decompression.
- Different algorithms for use of EUS-BD have been proposed, but none has been universally accepted. Therefore, any intervention for relieving biliary obstruction should depend largely on the particular clinical context.
- For patients with advanced or decompensated liver disease who are at higher risk for surgical complications and require nonoperative interventions for acute cholecystitis, EUS-GB can be considered (compared to LC, PC, or ETP).

DISCLOSURE

There was no grant support or other funding sources involved in the conduction, research, or writing of this article. The authors disclose no financial or commercial arrangements or conflicts of interest related to the research or assistance with article preparation.

REFERENCES

1. Enochsson L, Swahn F, Arnelo U, et al. Nationwide, population-based data from 11,074 ERCP procedures from the Swedish Registry for gallstone surgery and ERCP. Gastrointest Endosc 2010;72(6). https://doi.org/10.1016/j.gie.2010.07.047.
2. Mutneja HR, Vohra I, Go A, et al. Temporal trends and mortality of post-ERCP pancreatitis in the United States: a nationwide analysis. Endoscopy 2021;53(4):357–66.
3. Bailey AA, Bourke MJ, Williams SJ, et al. A prospective randomized trial of cannulation technique in ERCP: Effects on technical success and post-ERCP pancreatitis. Endoscopy 2008;40(4):296–301.
4. Halttunen J, Meisner S, Aabakken L, et al. Difficult cannulation as defined by a prospective study of the Scandinavian association for Digestive endoscopy (SADE) in 907 ERCPs. Scand J Gastroenterol 2014;49(6):752–8.

5. Dhindsa BS, Mashiana HS, Dhaliwal A, et al. EUS-guided biliary drainage: a systematic review and meta-analysis. Endosc Ultrasound 2020;9(2):101–9.

6. Moss A, Morris E, Mac Mathuna P. Palliative biliary stents for obstructing pancreatic carcinoma. In: Mac Mathuna P, editor. Cochrane Database of systematic reviews. John Wiley & Sons, Ltd; 2006. https://doi.org/10.1002/14651858. CD004200.pub2.

7. El Chafic AH, Shah JN. Advances in biliary access. Curr Gastroenterol Rep 2020; 22(12). https://doi.org/10.1007/s11894-020-00800-3.

8. Pécsi D, Farkas N, Hegyi P, et al. Transpancreatic sphincterotomy is effective and safe in expert hands on the short term. Dig Dis Sci 2019;64(9):2429–44.

9. Krishnamoorthi R, Jayaraj M, Kozarek R. Endoscopic stents for the biliary tree and Pancreas. Curr Treat Options Gastroenterol 2017;15(3):397–415.

10. Edlund G, Ljungdahl M. Acute cholecystitis in the elderly. Am J Surg 1990;159(4). https://doi.org/10.1016/S0002-9610(05)81285-1.

11. Lee SS, Park DH, Hwang CY, et al. EUS-guided transmural cholecystostomy as rescue management for acute cholecystitis in elderly or high-risk patients: a prospective feasibility study. Gastrointest Endosc 2007;66(5):1008–12.

12. Gomi H, Solomkin JS, Schlossberg D, et al. Tokyo Guidelines 2018: antimicrobial therapy for acute cholangitis and cholecystitis. J Hepatobiliary Pancreat Sci 2018;25(1):3–16.

13. Hatzidakis AA, Prassopoulos P, Petinarakis I, et al. Acute cholecystitis in high-risk patients: percutaneous cholecystostomy vs conservative treatment. Eur Radiol 2002;12(7):1778–84.

14. AYB T. Outcomes and limitations in EUS-guided gallbladder drainage. Endosc Ultrasound 2019;8(Suppl 1). https://doi.org/10.4103/EUS.EUS_49_19.

15. Teoh AYB, Kitano M, Itoi T, et al. Endosonography-guided gallbladder drainage versus percutaneous cholecystostomy in very high-risk surgical patients with acute cholecystitis: an international randomised multicentre controlled superiority trial (DRAC 1). Gut 2020;69(6):1085–91.

16. Luk SWY, Irani S, Krishnamoorthi R, et al. Endoscopic ultrasound-guided gallbladder drainage versus percutaneous cholecystostomy for high risk surgical patients with acute cholecystitis: a systematic review and meta-Analysis. Endoscopy 2019;51(8):722–32.

17. Giovannini M, Moutardier V, Pesenti C, et al. Endoscopic ultrasound-guided bilioduodenal anastomosis: a new technique for biliary drainage. Endoscopy 2001; 33(10):898–900.

18. Miller CS, Barkun AN, Martel M, et al. Endoscopic ultrasound-guided biliary drainage for distal malignant obstruction: a systematic review and meta-analysis of randomized trials. Endosc Int Open 2019;07(11):E1563–73.

19. Iwashita T, Doi S, Yasuda I. Endoscopic ultrasound-guided biliary drainage: a review. Clin J Gastroenterol 2014;7(2):94–102.

20. Vila JJ, Pérez-Miranda M, Vazquez-Sequeiros E, et al. Initial experience with EUS-guided cholangiopancreatography for biliary and pancreatic duct drainage: a Spanish national survey. Gastrointest Endosc 2012;76(6):1133–41.

21. Attasaranya S, Netinasunton N, Jongboonyanuparp T, et al. The spectrum of endoscopic ultrasound intervention in biliary diseases: a single center's experience in 31 cases. Gastroenterol Res Pract 2012;2012. https://doi.org/10.1155/2012/680753.

22. Wang K, Zhu J, Xing L, et al. Assessment of efficacy and safety of EUS-guided biliary drainage: a systematic review. Gastrointest Endosc 2016;83(6):1218–27.

23. Hedjoudje A, Sportes A, Grabar S, et al. Outcomes of endoscopic ultrasound-guided biliary drainage: a systematic review and meta-analysis. United Eur Gastroenterol J 2019;7(1):60–8.

24. Saad WEA, Wallace MJ, Wojak JC, et al. Quality improvement guidelines for percutaneous transhepatic Cholangiography, biliary drainage, and percutaneous cholecystostomy. J Vasc Interv Radiol 2010;21(6):789–95.

25. Sharaiha RZ, Khan MA, Kamal F, et al. Efficacy and safety of EUS-guided biliary drainage in comparison with percutaneous biliary drainage when ERCP fails: a systematic review and meta-analysis. Gastrointest Endosc 2017;85(5):904–14.

26. Ulusakarya A, Teyar N, Karaboué A, et al. Patient-tailored FOLFIRINOX as first line treatment of patients with advanced pancreatic adenocarcinoma. Medicine (Baltimore) 2019;98(16):e15341.

27. Born P, Rösch T, Triptrap A, et al. Long-term results of percutaneous transhepatic biliary drainage for benign and malignant bile duct strictures. Scand J Gastroenterol 1998;33(5):544–9.

28. Kakked G, Salameh H, Cheesman A, et al. Primary EUS-guided biliary drainage versus ERCP drainage for the management of malignant biliary obstruction: a systematic review and meta-analysis. Endosc Ultrasound 2020;9(5):298–307.

29. Han SY, Kim SO, So H, et al. EUS-guided biliary drainage versus ERCP for first-line palliation of malignant distal biliary obstruction: a systematic review and meta-analysis. Sci Rep 2019;9(1):1–9.

30. Paik WH, Lee TH, Park DH, et al. EUS-guided biliary drainage versus ERCP for the primary palliation of malignant biliary obstruction: a multicenter randomized clinical trial. Am J Gastroenterol 2018;113(7):987–97.

31. Mohan BP, Khan SR, Trakroo S, et al. Endoscopic ultrasound-guided gallbladder drainage, transpapillary drainage, or percutaneous drainage in high risk acute cholecystitis patients: a systematic review and comparative meta-analysis. Endoscopy 2020;52(2):96–106.

32. Podboy A, Yuan J, Stave CD, et al. Comparison of EUS-guided endoscopic transpapillary and percutaneous gallbladder drainage for acute cholecystitis: a systematic review with network meta-analysis. Gastrointest Endosc 2021;93(4):797–804.e1.

33. Teoh AYB, Leung CH, Tam PTH, et al. EUS-guided gallbladder drainage versus laparoscopic cholecystectomy for acute cholecystitis: a propensity score analysis with 1-year follow-up data. Gastrointest Endosc 2021;93(3):577–83.

34. Chan SM, Teoh AYB, Yip HC, et al. Feasibility of per-oral cholecystoscopy and advanced gallbladder interventions after EUS-guided gallbladder stenting (with video). Gastrointest Endosc 2017;85(6):1225–32.

35. Veitch AM, Baglin TP, Gershlick AH, et al. Guidelines for the management of anticoagulant and antiplatelet therapy in patients undergoing endoscopic procedures. Gut 2008;57(9):1322–9.

36. Fujimoto K, Fujishiro M, Kato M, et al. Guidelines for gastroenterological endoscopy in patients undergoing antithrombotic treatment. Dig Endosc 2014;26(1):1–14.

37. Okuno N, Hara K, Mizuno N, et al. Outcomes of endoscopic ultrasound-guided biliary drainage in patients undergoing antithrombotic therapy. Clin Endosc 2021. https://doi.org/10.5946/ce.2020.194.

38. Vozzo CF, Simons-Linares CR, Abou Saleh M, et al. Safety of EUS-guided gallbladder drainage using a lumen-apposing metal stent in patients requiring anticoagulation. VideoGIE 2020;5(10):500–3.e1.

39. Anderloni A, Attili F, Sferrazza A, et al. EUS-guided gallbladder drainage using a lumen-apposing self-expandable metal stent in patients with coagulopathy or anticoagulation therapy: a case series. Endosc Int Open 2017;05(11):E1100–3.

40. Krishnamoorthi R, Dasari CS, Thoguluva Chandrasekar V, et al. Effectiveness and safety of EUS-guided choledochoduodenostomy using lumen-apposing metal stents (LAMS): a systematic review and meta-analysis. Surg Endosc 2020; 34(7):2866–77.

41. Tringali A, Hassan C, Rota M, et al. Covered vsuncovered self-expandable metal stents for malignant distal biliary strictures: a systematic review and meta-analysis. Endoscopy 2018;50(6):631–41.

42. Kalva NR, Vanar V, Forcione D, et al. Efficacy and safety of lumen apposing self-expandable metal stents for EUS guided cholecystostomy: a meta-analysis and systematic review. Can J Gastroenterol Hepatol 2018;2018. https://doi.org/10.1155/2018/7070961.

43. Anderloni A, Fugazza A, Troncone E, et al. Single-stage EUS-guided choledochoduodenostomy using a lumen-apposing metal stent for malignant distal biliary obstruction. Gastrointest Endosc 2019;89(1):69–76.

44. Brimhall B, Han S, Tatman PD, et al. Increased incidence of Pseudoaneurysm bleeding with lumen-apposing metal stents compared to double-pigtail plastic stents in patients with Peripancreatic fluid collections. Clin Gastroenterol Hepatol 2018;16(9):1521–8.

45. Garcia-Sumalla A, Loras C, Guarner-Argente C, et al. Is a coaxial plastic stent within a lumen-apposing metal stent useful for the management of distal malignant biliary obstruction? Surg Endosc 2021. https://doi.org/10.1007/s00464-021-08435-9.

46. Ogura T, Nishioka N, Yamada M, et al. Comparison study between double bare covered and fully covered metal stent during endoscopic ultrasound-guided choledochoduodenostomy (with video). Dig Dis 2021;39(2):165–70.

47. Varadarajulu S, Hawes RH. EUS-guided biliary drainage: Taxing and not ready. Gastrointest Endosc 2013;78(5):742–3.

48. Park DH, Lee TH, Paik WH, et al. Feasibility and safety of a novel dedicated device for one-step EUS-guided biliary drainage: a randomized trial. J Gastroenterol Hepatol 2015;30(10):1461–6.

49. Conio M, Demarquay JF, De Luca L, et al. Endoscopic treatment of pancreaticobiliary malignancies. Crit Rev Oncol Hematol 2001;37(2):127–35.

50. Bang JY, Navaneethan U, Hasan M, et al. Stent placement by EUS or ERCP for primary biliary decompression in pancreatic cancer: a randomized trial (with videos). Gastrointest Endosc 2018;88(1):9–17.

51. Khan MA, Akbar A, Baron TH, et al. Endoscopic ultrasound-guided biliary drainage: a systematic review and meta-analysis. Dig Dis Sci 2016;61(3):684–703.

52. Tyberg A, Desai AP, Kumta NA, et al. EUS-guided biliary drainage after failed ERCP: a novel algorithm individualized based on patient anatomy. Gastrointest Endosc 2016;84(6):941–6.

53. Khoo S, Do NT, Kongkam P. Efficacy and safety of EUS biliary drainage in malignant distal and hilar biliary obstruction: a comprehensive review of literature and algorithm. Endosc Ultrasound 2020;9(6):369.

Endoscopic Ultrasound for the Diagnosis and Staging of Biliary Malignancy

Martin Coronel, MD, Jeffrey H. Lee, MD, MPH,
Emmanuel Coronel, MD*

KEYWORDS

- Biliary strictures • Cholangiocarcinoma • Endoscopic ultrasound
- Fine-needle aspiration

KEY POINTS

- Endoscopic ultrasound is safe and effective in the diagnosis of cholangiocarcinoma.
- For the diagnosis of distal biliary strictures, endoscopic ultrasound (EUS) should be considered first-line and, if necessary, combined with endoscopic retrograde cholangiopancreatography (ERCP) for tissue acquisition.
- For the diagnosis of perihilar strictures, ERCP should be considered first line. In addition, EUS can be used to assess lymph nodes, which is helpful not only for diagnosis but also for staging purposes. However, EUS-fine-needle aspiration (EUS-FNA) of the primary tumor should be avoided due to the risk of seeding.
- A repeat EUS or ERCP should be considered if clinically indicated in patients with previously negative tissue sampling and high suspicion of cancer.

CHOLANGIOCARCINOMA: DEFINITION, BASIC PRINCIPLES, AND CHALLENGES

Cholangiocarcinoma (CCA) is the most common neoplasm of the biliary tract and this is a malignancy of aggressive behavior arising from the biliary epithelium and creating a desmoplastic stroma resulting in biliary strictures. By location, it can be divided into intrahepatic and extrahepatic. Extrahepatic tumors can be further divided into perihilar and distal **Fig. 1**. This is an important distinction because the biological behavior and prognosis differ depending on the tumor's location in the biliary tree, dictating a different diagnostic and treatment approach.

Most CCAs are extrahepatic, accounting for approximately 80% of CCA cases diagnosed in the United States. The highest global incidence of CCA comes from Thailand and this is mainly attributed to liver fluke infections, which are endemic in Southeast Asia. In the western world, age-adjusted incidence rates of intrahepatic CCA have

Department of Gastroenterology, Hepatology, and Nutrition, The University of Texas, MD Anderson Cancer Center, 1515 Holcombe Boulevard, Unit 1466, Houston, TX 77030, USA
* Corresponding author.
E-mail address: ecoronel@mdanderson.org

Clin Liver Dis 26 (2022) 115–125
https://doi.org/10.1016/j.cld.2021.08.010
1089-3261/22/© 2021 Elsevier Inc. All rights reserved.

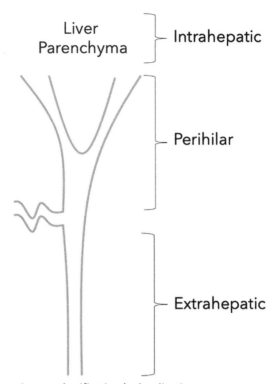

Fig. 1. Cholangiocarcinoma, classification by localization.

increased, whereas the incidence of extrahepatic CCA has followed a stable to decreasing trend. Significant risk factors for CCA in the west are the presence of primary sclerosing cholangitis (PSC), inflammatory bowel disease, obesity, diabetes, viral hepatitis, cirrhosis, biliary lithiasis, and biliary cysts.[1,2]

CCA carries a poor prognosis, even in resectable patients with a 5-year survival rate ranging from 10% to 40% and a recurrence rate of 50% to 70% after surgical resection.[3]

Establishing a diagnosis of CCA remains a challenge, as diagnostic tissue sampling of biliary strictures can yield benign pathology in 30% and indeterminate results in 20% of cases.[4] Although a tissue diagnosis is critical for patients before initiating chemotherapy or radiation, it is not mandatory for surgical resection or transplantation. This is another important distinction, as most patients with biliary malignancy present with unresectable or metastatic disease and are candidates for life-prolonging treatments.[3]

Recent advances in endoscopic technologies have paved the way for significant improvements in securing a tissue diagnosis in CCA. Traditionally, endoscopic retrograde cholangiopancreatography (ERCP)-based techniques (biliary brushings, forceps biopsies, cholangioscopy) have been used for the tissue acquisition of biliary strictures and suspected CCA. However, in the last few years, endoscopic ultrasound (EUS) has been increasingly used as an effective diagnostic tool. It provides high-quality images of the bile duct and surrounding structures such as the pancreas, liver, hepatic hilum, vasculature, and lymph nodes. Although the radial echoendoscope provides cross-sectional, 360-degree purely diagnostic images, the linear array echoendoscope provides sagittal images parallel to the axis of the endoscope and is equipped with an accessory channel allowing for tissue sampling in the same plane of view.

Whereas ERCP and EUS-based tissue acquisition techniques are complementary, we will discuss the importance of EUS in the diagnosis and staging of biliary malignancy in this chapter.

ENDOSCOPIC ULTRASOUND AND TISSUE SAMPLING IN BILIARY MALIGNANCY

EUS provides excellent images of the pancreas and distal bile duct, making it the preferred technique to acquire tissue from pancreatic lesions, and more recently, biliary strictures, masses, and lymph nodes. In one of the first case series published in 2000, the authors analyzed the outcomes of EUS and fine-needle aspiration (FNA) in 10 patients who had previously negative brushings via ERCP despite high suspicion of perihilar CCA. Adequate material was obtained in 9 patients, establishing a diagnosis of CCA in 7 patients and hepatocellular carcinoma (HCC) in one. One patient had a false negative FNA result, and 2 patients were found to have metastatic loco-regional lymph nodes.[5] The same group published results of a larger study that included 44 patients. The authors found that EUS-FNA for biliary strictures had a sensitivity of 91% and specificity of 89%, and more importantly, it changed surgical decision-making in 27 out of 44 cases.[6] Other studies confirmed similar findings demonstrating that EUS-FNA for suspected CCA can prevent unnecessary surgery in patients with unresectable disease or benign disease, yet facilitating surgery when other diagnostic modalities could not secure a cancer diagnosis.[7]

As aforementioned, CCA is associated with poor prognosis, and only a small fraction of patients are candidates for surgical resection or transplantation. The Mayo Clinic developed the first protocol for liver transplantation in patients with perihilar CCA and this process involves an extensive preoperative evaluation. If a candidate is eligible, they will undergo neoadjuvant chemotherapy, radiation, and an exploratory laparotomy to assess resectability and metastasis. This highly selective treatment algorithm showed better survival outcomes and lower recurrence rates of liver transplantation when compared with resection alone. In 2002, Mayo Clinic included EUS-FNA into the algorithm, with the purpose to evaluate regional lymph nodes before neoadjuvant treatment. In a study published in 2008, authors from the same institution assessed the outcomes of preoperative EUS-FNA in 47 patients who were transplant candidates. EUS-FNA detected nodal metastasis in 17% of the cases, precluding transplantation, and in 20 out of 22 cases, the node-negative disease was confirmed by exploratory laparotomy. No EUS imaging features of the lymph nodes were found to be predictive of malignancy.

In patients who are liver transplant candidates, EUS-FNA of the primary lesion should not be performed due to the risk of needle tract seeding..[8–10] In a study of 191 patients who underwent transplant evaluation for locally advanced (unresectable) perihilar CCA, including 16 patients who underwent transperitoneal FNA of a primary tumor (13 percutaneous, 3 EUS guided), peritoneal metastasis was discovered at operative staging in 83% (5/6) of patients with confirmed CCA compared with only 8% (14/175) of patients who were not biopsied ($P = .0097$).

Since the development of this algorithm, most institutions that offer liver transplant as a treatment option for perihilar CCA considers percutaneous, laparoscopic, or EUS-guided biopsies of the primary tumor a contraindication for transplantation.

Although EUS-FNA of CCA is an absolute contraindication for transplantation, it is not an absolute contraindication for surgical resection, mainly when the tumor is in the distal bile duct. In a retrospective study of 150 cases with confirmed CCA, 61 underwent preoperative EUS-FNA. The authors found that the performance of EUS-FNA with a median number of 5 passes had no impact on overall or progression-free survival. In addition, they found that small tumor size and the absence of nodal disease were correlated with improved survival outcomes, and this is essential information that can be obtained by EUS-imaging and correlated with cross-sectional imaging studies.[11]

In a meta-analysis of 20 studies, including 957 patients, EUS-FNA was found to be highly accurate for the diagnosis of malignant biliary strictures, showing a sensitivity of 80% (95% confidence interval [CI]: 74%–86%), specificity of 97% (95% CI: 94%–99%) with a pooled diagnostic odds ratio (OR) of 70.53% (95% CI: 38.62%–128.82%), and an area under the receiver-operating characteristic curve of 0.97, demonstrating that the performance of EUS-FNA as a diagnostic tool for malignant biliary strictures is excellent.[12] A meta-analysis of 10 studies demonstrated that the incremental benefit of EUS-FNA in patients who had undergone previous nondiagnostic ERCP with brushings was 14% (95% CI: 7%–20%). Furthermore, a meta-analysis of 6 studies including 497 patients who underwent the same session EUS and ERCP tissue sampling showed that the sensitivity and accuracy of EUS alone versus EUS combined with ERCP were 76% and 94.5% versus 86% and 96.5%, respectively,[13] suggesting that the same session EUS and ERCP should be considered when necessary and that these diagnostic methods are complementary to each other. An example of EUS-FNA of the distal bile duct, combined with ERCP with brushings and wire-guided biopsies, is depicted in **Fig. 2**A.

ENDOSCOPIC ULTRASOUND AND ITS ROLE IN THE STAGING OF BILIARY MALIGNANCY

Accurate staging of CCA is critical, as it provides a blueprint for treatment options being curative in early-stage disease versus life-prolonging in advanced stages. Therefore, the first step in staging should be obtaining high-quality cross-sectional imaging, as it provides crucial tumor-related information, such as localization, local tumor extension, vascular involvement, nodal status, and detection of distant metastasis. This can be in the form of multiphasic contrast-enhanced computed tomography (CT) or contrast-enhanced magnetic resonance imaging/cholangiopancreatography (MRI/MRCP), each one of them having its advantages and disadvantages.[14] Depending on the localization of the tumor and additional information that may be required, EUS can be used as an adjunct to complete the staging workup.

In a large, single-center retrospective study of 228 patients with biliary strictures and 81 patients with a confirmed CCA diagnosis, the authors determined that EUS had a significant advantage in tumor detection than CT with a sensitivity of 53% and specificity of 97% in detecting unresectability. Features of unresectability by EUS were listed as: the presence of noncontiguous liver nodules suspicious for metastasis, ascites, detection of malignant appearing, nonregional lymph nodes, tumor involvement of the main portal vein (PV), bilateral PV branches, and hepatic artery.[15]

In a recently published study, which analyzed the outcomes of 157 patients with confirmed CCA, EUS found more metastatic lymph nodes than cross-sectional imaging, and encountering a metastatic node was correlated with worse survival outcomes and an increased risk of death.[16] In a study of 52 patients with pancreatobiliary cancers and enlarged peri-aortic lymph nodes found on imaging, EUS-FNA was highly accurate, making a correct diagnosis of malignancy in 95.2% of cases, than positron

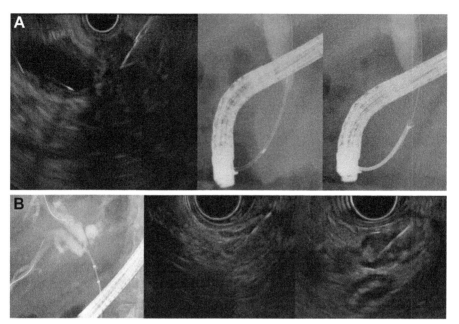

Fig. 2. (A) EUS imaging of a distal biliary stricture and FNA (*left*). Fluoroscopic imaging of ERCP and biliary brushings (*middle*) and wire-guided biopsy forceps (*right*). (B) Fluoroscopic image of a perihilar cholangiocarcinoma (*left*). EUS-FNA of a periportal lymph node (*middle*) and a gastrohepatic lymph node (*right*) were performed for staging purposes.

emission tomography (PET)/CT in 57.1% of cases.[17] An example of EUS-FNA for locoregional lymphadenopathy and staging purposes is depicted in **Fig. 2**B.

DIAGNOSTIC APPROACH TO BILIARY STRICTURES AND SUSPECTED BILIARY MALIGNANCY

A diagnostic approach algorithm followed in our practice is summarized in **Fig. 3**, which should be adjusted to individual practice, available resources, and on a case-by-case basis. This algorithm starts by identifying patients with suspected biliary strictures and recommends obtaining high-quality cross-sectional imaging and laboratory studies. IgG-4 levels should be obtained in patients with distal biliary strictures and the absence of a mass. If elevated, a trial of steroids can be considered IgG-4 related sclerosing cholangitis can present with biliary stenosis. Even in cases with normal IgG-4 serologies, the possibility of this disease should not be dismissed entirely, as 30% of cases of autoimmune cholangiopathy can be IgG-4 negative. In this instance, findings such as histology, imaging, serology, other organ involvement, and response to steroids (HISORt criteria) can be used to establish a diagnosis.[18] In patients with distal biliary strictures, EUS should be the first diagnostic modality used to obtain tissue. When necessary, ERCP should be used as an adjunct diagnostic tool before biliary stenting. For perihilar strictures, however, ERCP should be the first diagnostic modality. EUS can be used as an adjunct when ERCP is inconclusive; caution must be exercised as EUS-FNA of the primary tumor is contraindicated in patients with perihilar

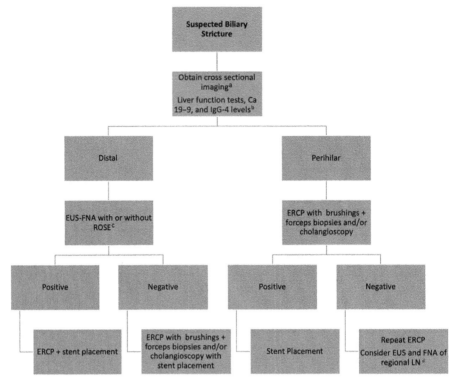

Fig. 3. Algorithm - Diagnostic Approach for Suspected Biliary Strictures [a]Cross-sectional imaging should be of high quality; ideally, multiphasic contrast-enhanced CT imaging or contrast-enhanced MRI. [b]IgG-4 levels should be obtained in distal biliary strictures without a pancreatic mass. A high IgG-4 level may indicate autoimmune cholangiopathy; a trial of high-dose steroids can be considered a diagnostic/therapeutic intervention. [c]In our institution, rapid onsite cytology evaluation by a cytology attending is available and this allows ERCP in the same endoscopic session of EUS or repeat sampling with a different technique during ERCP. If performed in a separate session, repeat procedures should be performed early to avoid treatment delays, ideally within 4 weeks after the index procedure. [d]EUS-FNA of the primary tumor should be avoided in perihilar cholangiocarcinoma as it is an absolute contraindication for transplantation. However, if the patient is not a transplant candidate, EUS-FNA of the primary tumor may be considered in select cases and after multidisciplinary discussion. EUS, endoscopic ultrasound; ERCP, endoscopic retrograde cholangiopancreatography; FNA, fine-needle aspiration; LNs, lymph nodes.

CCA who are potential transplant candidates. As transplant candidacy may not be defined at this stage of the workup, we recommend avoiding EUS-FNA of the primary tumor. However, EUS can still be performed for loco-regional staging and evaluation of enlarged lymph nodes. Furthermore, EUS can be of value in patients with intrahepatic CCA, particularly in surgical candidates, as nodal staging is an important prognostic indicator. In patients with inconclusive results and high suspicion of cancer, a repeat EUS-FNA or ERCP with tissue sampling should be strongly considered, particularly in centers of excellence, as it may improve diagnostic outcomes.[19–21] If clinically appropriate, this should be performed early to avoid delays in treatment, ideally within 4 weeks after the index procedure.

ANCILLARY TECHNIQUES, NEW TECHNOLOGIES, AND FUTURE DIRECTIONS

Multiple needle sizes and designs are available for EUS-guided tissue sampling. Most published data show no statistically significant difference in diagnostic performance among 19-, 20-, 22-, and 25-gauge needles.[22] A study comparing EUS-guided fine-needle core biopsies (FNB) of biliary lesions to cholangioscopy-guided biopsies showed that both methods were highly accurate (more than 90%). A 22-gauge FNB needle with a core trap cutout was used in this study; however, safety could not be assessed as complications were not reported..[23] Most of the data comparing the accuracy of needle sizes and designs come from sampling solid pancreatic lesions. No significant difference between different needle sizes or designs was encountered in a meta-analysis, but these estimates were of low confidence.[24] Due to the rigidity of 19-gauge needles, we prefer to use 25-gauge FNA needles as first-line and 22-gauge FNA needles or FNB needles as a second line in cases whereby samples are not adequate.

Rapid onsite evaluation (ROSE) provides immediate intraprocedural feedback. In some studies, it has been shown to increase the diagnostic yield of EUS-FNA, improve sample adequacy, and decrease the number of needle passes.[25–27] Although ROSE may reduce the number of repeat procedures[21] and avoid delays, it is expensive, time-consuming, and not widely available. In a multicenter, randomized trial, the diagnostic accuracy of FNB needles alone was noninferior to EUS-FNA with ROSE and had a comparable cost.[28] This may be a good alternative for endoscopy practices whereby ROSE is not available.

Besides conventional cytology, fluorescence in situ hybridization (FISH) can be considered an ancillary technique. In a study of 250 patients who underwent EUS-guided sampling of suspected malignancy of different anatomic sites, the combination of these diagnostic techniques improved the sensitivity of cytology alone.[29] EUS-FNA can also provide samples that can be used for next-generation sequencing (NGS). For example, in a study of 21 patients with carcinoma of the biliary tree, adequate samples for genetic analysis were obtained in 20 out of 21 patients. The authors obtained samples using 22-gauge or 25-gauge needles and used ROSE and refrigeration before genetic analysis.[30] In patients with pancreatobiliary cancers, EUS can be used to obtain portal venous blood samples and circulating tumor cells (CTCs) can be measured as a biomarker that may predict solid tumor burden and survival.[31] The use of these technologies should be explored ideally under a research protocol, and safety considerations should be put in place as additional needle passes may be needed.

Intraductal ultrasound (IDUS) of the biliary tree can be performed using a dedicated wire-guided US catheter. The catheter can be introduced in the biliary tree using ERCP. This technology has been shown to help evaluate biliary strictures in patients who present without a mass on abdominal imaging. The use of IDUS in combination with ERCP increases the accuracy of ERCP, and it may help better characterize the lesion as patients with pancreatic parenchymal invasion when seen on IDUS, can undergo conventional EUS. In such cases, a pancreatic mass was found by EUS in more than 50% of patients.[32]

The use of artificial intelligence (AI) has sparked interest in the scientific community. Through the application of convolutional neural networks (CNN), medical images can be analyzed, and these algorithms can be trained to detect cancer with higher accuracy than experts. Although in very early stages and not yet studied for biliary malignancy, EUS images have been used to build CNNs to recognize pancreatic lesions, focal liver lesions, and autoimmune pancreatitis with excellent diagnostic performance.[33–35] This is an exciting new technology and its application could be beneficial in this challenging patient population.

SAFETY CONSIDERATIONS AND LIMITATIONS

EUS tissue acquisition of the bile duct has a favorable safety profile. In a meta-analysis of 497 patients, a total of 34 complications were reported in 6 studies. Although these complications were mostly minor, including cholangitis, pancreatitis, and mild bleeding episodes, one patient developed biliary peritonitis and died after surgery.[13] As mentioned above, EUS-FNA of the primary tumor should be avoided in patients with perihilar CCA due to the risk of needle tract seeding.[10]

Biliary stents may hinder EUS imaging as they cast an acoustic shadow that interferes with visualization. Data from cholangioscopy-guided biopsies show that the diagnostic yield of indeterminate biliary strictures in patients with PSC or previously placed biliary stents may be lower; this may also apply to EUS-guided biopsies.[36–38]

SUMMARY

EUS is a safe and effective tool in the diagnosis and staging of CCA. EUS should be considered first line in patients with distal strictures and an important adjunct for nodal staging in patients with perihilar or intrahepatic disease. Special caution should be exercised in patients with perihilar strictures, as EUS-guided biopsy of the primary tumor is an absolute contraindication for liver transplantation.

CLINICS CARE POINTS

- EUS is a safe and effective tool in the diagnosis and staging of CCA.
- Obtaining high-quality cross-sectional imaging is paramount and the location of the tumor dictates the diagnostic and therapeutic approach.
- EUS-FNA of distal biliary strictures should be considered first-line and ERCP as an adjunct because a combined approach may improve the diagnostic yield.
- ERCP-based tissue acquisition should be considered first line in perihilar CCA, and EUS-FNA of the primary tumor should be avoided.
- In patients with suspected perihilar CCA, EUS-guided lymph node biopsies should be considered for diagnostic and staging purposes.
- In patients who have a "negative" ERCP or EUS and a high suspicion of cancer, a repeat procedure should be considered, ideally at centers of excellence and within 4 weeks of the index procedure to avoid delays in treatment.

DISCLOSURE

Dr M. Coronel has no disclosures. Dr J.H. Lee has no disclosures. Dr E. Coronel is a consultant for Boston Scientific.

REFERENCES

1. Blechacz B. Cholangiocarcinoma: current knowledge and new developments. Gut Liver 2017;11(1):13–26.
2. Shaib YH, El-Serag HB, Davila JA, et al. Risk factors of intrahepatic cholangiocarcinoma in the United States: a case-control study. Gastroenterology 2005;128(3): 620–6.
3. Krampitz GW, Aloia TA. Staging of biliary and primary liver tumors: current recommendations and workup. Surg Oncol Clin N Am 2019;28(4):663–83.

4. Bowlus CL, Olson KA, Gershwin ME. Evaluation of indeterminate biliary strictures. Nat Rev Gastroenterol Hepatol 2016;13(1):28–37.

5. Fritscher-Ravens A, Broering DC, Sriram PV, et al. EUS-guided fine-needle aspiration cytodiagnosis of hilar cholangiocarcinoma: a case series. Gastrointest Endosc 2000;52(4):534–40.

6. Fritscher-Ravens A, Broering DC, Knoefel WT, et al. EUS-guided fine-needle aspiration of suspected hilar cholangiocarcinoma in potentially operable patients with negative brush cytology. Am J Gastroenterol 2004;99(1):45–51.

7. Eloubeidi MA, Chen VK, Jhala NC, et al. Endoscopic ultrasound-guided fine needle aspiration biopsy of suspected cholangiocarcinoma. Clin Gastroenterol Hepatol 2004;2(3):209–13.

8. Rea DJ, Heimbach JK, Rosen CB, et al. Liver transplantation with neoadjuvant chemoradiation is more effective than resection for hilar cholangiocarcinoma. Ann Surg 2005;242(3):451–8 [Discussion 458–61].

9. Gleeson FC, Rajan E, Levy MJ, et al. EUS-guided FNA of regional lymph nodes in patients with unresectable hilar cholangiocarcinoma. Gastrointest Endosc 2008; 67(3):438–43.

10. Gleeson FC, Lee JH, Dewitt JM. Tumor seeding associated with selected gastrointestinal endoscopic interventions. Clin Gastroenterol Hepatol 2018;16(9):1385–8.

11. El Chafic AH, Dewitt J, Leblanc JK, et al. Impact of preoperative endoscopic ultrasound-guided fine needle aspiration on postoperative recurrence and survival in cholangiocarcinoma patients. Endoscopy 2013;45(11):883–9.

12. Sadeghi A, Mohamadnejad M, Islami F, et al. Diagnostic yield of EUS-guided FNA for malignant biliary stricture: a systematic review and meta-analysis. Gastrointest Endosc 2016;83(2):290–8.e1.

13. de Moura DTH, Ryou M, de Moura EGH, et al. Endoscopic ultrasound-guided fine needle aspiration and endoscopic retrograde cholangiopancreatography-based tissue sampling in suspected malignant biliary strictures: a meta-analysis of same-session procedures. Clin Endosc 2020;53(4):417–28.

14. Buckholz AP, Brown RS Jr. Cholangiocarcinoma: diagnosis and management. Clin Liver Dis 2020;24(3):421–36.

15. Mohamadnejad M, DeWitt JM, Sherman S, et al. Role of EUS for preoperative evaluation of cholangiocarcinoma: a large single-center experience. Gastrointest Endosc 2011;73(1):71–8.

16. Malikowski T, Levy MJ, Gleeson FC, et al. Endoscopic ultrasound/fine needle aspiration is effective for lymph node staging in patients with cholangiocarcinoma. Hepatology 2020;72(3):940–8.

17. Kurita A, Kodama Y, Nakamoto Y, et al. Impact of EUS-FNA for preoperative para-aortic lymph node staging in patients with pancreatobiliary cancer. Gastrointest Endosc 2016;84(3):467–75.e1.

18. Chari ST. Diagnosis of autoimmune pancreatitis using its five cardinal features: introducing the Mayo Clinic's HISORt criteria. J Gastroenterol 2007;42(Suppl 18):39–41.

19. Yang X, Guo JF, Sun LQ, et al. Assessment of different modalities for repeated tissue acquisition in diagnosing malignant biliary strictures: a two-center retrospective study. J Dig Dis 2021;22(2):102–7.

20. DeWitt J, McGreevy K, Sherman S, et al. Utility of a repeated EUS at a tertiary-referral center. Gastrointest Endosc 2008;67(4):610–9.

21. Lisotti A, Frazzoni L, Fuccio L, et al. Repeat EUS-FNA of pancreatic masses after nondiagnostic or inconclusive results: systematic review and meta-analysis. Gastrointest Endosc 2020;91(6):1234–41.e4.

22. Jo JH, Cho CM, Jun JH, et al. Same-session endoscopic ultrasound-guided fine needle aspiration and endoscopic retrograde cholangiopancreatography-based tissue sampling in suspected malignant biliary obstruction: a multicenter experience. J Gastroenterol Hepatol 2019;34(4):799–805.

23. Lee YN, Moon JH, Choi HJ, et al. Tissue acquisition for diagnosis of biliary strictures using peroral cholangioscopy or endoscopic ultrasound-guided fine-needle aspiration. Endoscopy 2019;51(1):50–9.

24. Facciorusso A, Wani S, Triantafyllou K, et al. Comparative accuracy of needle sizes and designs for EUS tissue sampling of solid pancreatic masses: a network meta-analysis. Gastrointest Endosc 2019;90(6):893–903.e7.

25. Klapman JB, Logrono R, Dye CE, et al. Clinical impact of on-site cytopathology interpretation on endoscopic ultrasound-guided fine needle aspiration. Am J Gastroenterol 2003;98(6):1289–94.

26. Khoury T, Kadah A, Farraj M, et al. The role of rapid on-site evaluation on diagnostic accuracy of endoscopic ultrasound fine needle aspiration for pancreatic, submucosal upper gastrointestinal tract and adjacent lesions. Cytopathology 2019;30(5):499–503.

27. Matynia AP, Schmidt RL, Barraza G, et al. Impact of rapid on-site evaluation on the adequacy of endoscopic-ultrasound guided fine-needle aspiration of solid pancreatic lesions: a systematic review and meta-analysis. J Gastroenterol Hepatol 2014;29(4):697–705.

28. Chen YI, Chatterjee A, Berger R, et al. Endoscopic ultrasound (EUS)-guided fine needle biopsy alone vs. EUS-guided fine needle aspiration with rapid onsite evaluation in pancreatic lesions: a multicenter randomized trial. Endoscopy 2021. [Epub ahead of print].

29. Levy MJ, Oberg TN, Campion MB, et al. Comparison of methods to detect neoplasia in patients undergoing endoscopic ultrasound-guided fine-needle aspiration. Gastroenterology 2012;142(5):1112–21.e2.

30. Hirata K, Kuwatani M, Suda G, et al. A novel approach for the genetic analysis of biliary tract cancer Specimens obtained through endoscopic ultrasound-guided fine needle aspiration using targeted amplicon sequencing. Clin Transl Gastroenterol 2019;10(3):e00022.

31. Catenacci DV, Chapman CG, Xu P, et al. Acquisition of portal venous circulating tumor cells from patients with pancreaticobiliary cancers by endoscopic ultrasound. Gastroenterology 2015;149(7):1794–803.e4.

32. Stavropoulos S, Larghi A, Verna E, et al. Intraductal ultrasound for the evaluation of patients with biliary strictures and no abdominal mass on computed tomography. Endoscopy 2005;37(8):715–21.

33. Marya NB, Powers PD, Chari ST, et al. Utilisation of artificial intelligence for the development of an EUS-convolutional neural network model trained to enhance the diagnosis of autoimmune pancreatitis. Gut 2021;70(7):1335–44.

34. Marya NB, Powers PD, Fujii-Lau L, et al. Application of artificial intelligence using a novel EUS-based convolutional neural network model to identify and distinguish benign and malignant hepatic masses. Gastrointest Endosc 2021;93(5):1121–30.e1.

35. Săftoiu A, Vilmann P, Gorunescu F, et al. Efficacy of an artificial neural network-based approach to endoscopic ultrasound elastography in diagnosis of focal pancreatic masses. Clin Gastroenterol Hepatol 2012;10(1):84–90.e1.

36. Bekkali NLH, Nayar MK, Leeds JS, et al. Impact of metal and plastic stents on endoscopic ultrasound-guided aspiration cytology and core histology of head of pancreas masses. Endoscopy 2019;51(11):1044–50.

37. de Vries AB, van der Heide F, Ter Steege RWF, et al. Limited diagnostic accuracy and clinical impact of single-operator peroral cholangioscopy for indeterminate biliary strictures. Endoscopy 2020;52(2):107–14.
38. Raine T, Thomas JP, Brais R, et al. Test performance and predictors of accuracy of endoscopic ultrasound-guided fine-needle aspiration for diagnosing biliary strictures or masses. Endosc Int Open 2020;8(11):E1537–44.

Endoscopic Ultrasound-Guided Liver Biopsy

Ishaan K. Madhok, MD[a], Nasim Parsa, MD[b], Jose M. Nieto, DO[c],*

KEYWORDS

- Endoscopic ultrasound-guided liver biopsy • Fine needle biopsy
- Fine needle aspiration • Core biopsy

KEY POINTS

- Endoscopic ultrasound-guided liver biopsy (EUS-LB) has emerged as a minimally invasive alternative approach for liver tissue acquisition with comparable diagnostic yield to percutaneous and trans-jugular approaches, and lower rate of complication.
- The ability to obtain bilobar biopsies can decrease the sampling error during EUS-LB.
- The novel 19-gauge core needle has been shown to be superior to the other needles for liver tissue acquisition.
- The wet suction technique provides superior tissue samples compared with the dry suction, as heparin can prevent blood clotting within the needle lumen.
- Further large, randomized trials are needed for procedural standardization.

INTRODUCTION

The increasing incidence of metabolic-associated fatty liver disease (MAFLD) and its relationship with cirrhosis and liver failure has brought attention to the importance of the accurate staging of liver fibrosis. Recently, there has been increased enthusiasm for noninvasive tests to assess liver fibrosis such as ultrasound elastography and serologic analysis. However, liver biopsy remains the gold standard diagnostic test for most of the focal and parenchymal liver diseases.[1] Liver biopsy has an important diagnostic role in selected parenchymal liver diseases such as autoimmune hepatitis and infiltrative liver disease, and in some cases, it helps clinicians elucidate between overlapping diagnoses. Traditionally, percutaneous (PC-LB), trans-jugular (TJ-LB), and surgical approaches have been used to acquire liver tissue samples. Endoscopic ultrasound-guided liver biopsy (EUS-LB) was first described in 2007 by Abraham Matthews.[2] Since then, the EUS-LB technique has evolved as an effective alternative to traditional methods in the diagnosis and staging of focal and parenchymal liver diseases. To

[a] Department of Internal Medicine, University of Florida, 1600 SW Archer Road, Room 4102, Gainesville, Fl, 32610-0277, USA; [b] Division of Gastroenterology and Hepatology, Mayo Clinic, 5777 E Mayo Blvd, Phoenix, Arizona 85054, USA; [c] Advanced Therapeutic Endoscopy Center, Borland Groover, 4336 Coastal Hwy, St. Augustine, FL 32084, USA
* Corresponding author.
E-mail address: drjnieto@gmail.com

Clin Liver Dis 26 (2022) 127–138
https://doi.org/10.1016/j.cld.2021.09.002
1089-3261/22/© 2021 Elsevier Inc. All rights reserved.
liver.theclinics.com

date, several studies have evaluated the diagnostic yield and safety profile of the EUS-LB. EUS-LB has shown to produce excellent histologic yield based on liver society guideline requirements for parameters used in assessing histologic yield which include the number of complete portal tracts (CPTs), sample size, intact specimen length (ISL), and total specimen length (TSL).[3]

EUS-LB has several advantages over the traditional liver biopsy methods (**Table 1**): it provides simultaneous access to both liver lobes which increases sampling accuracy while minimizing sampling error.[4,5] EUS-LB has the advantage of detecting smaller lesions (<10 mm) which can play an important role in patients being

Table 1
Comparison of minimally invasive liver biopsy techniques

	Advantages	Disadvantages
EUS-LB	• Can be performed simultaneously with other endoscopic procedures • Bilobar access allows for greater sampling • Real-time image guidance allows for avoiding critical structures • Body habitus does not affect procedure technical success • Early data show portal gradient pressures can be measured • May allow for better visualization of lesions for targeted liver biopsy • Allow for better evaluation of surrounding anatomy	• Costly as a procedure performed in absence of other indication for endoscopy • Requires the most expertise • Increased risk of bleeding due to requiring capsule puncture. May not be suitable if significant coagulopathy present • Unnecessary risks of anesthesia if no other need for deep sedation
PCN-LB	• Widely accessible • Cost-effective • Does not require deep sedation	• Subject to sampling variability • Cannot be performed if significant ascites • Body habitus can be technically limiting • Cannot measure portal pressure gradients • If using CT, lose real-time imaging capabilities to avoid damaging critical structures and cause radiation exposure • Increased risk of bleeding due to requiring capsular puncture. Not suitable if significant coagulopathy present. • Limited view of surrounding anatomy
TJ-LB	• Can obtain portal pressure gradient • Does not require capsular puncture so preferred in patients with significant coagulopathy • Body habitus is not as limiting a factor to technical success as in PCN • Can be performed in presence of significant ascites • Does not require deep sedation	• Requires technical expertise of interventional radiologist • Cannot obtain the biopsy of focal hepatic lesions • Subject to sampling variability • Limited view of surrounding anatomy

Abbreviations: EUS-LB, endoscopic ultrasound-guided liver biopsy; PCN-LB, percutaneous liver biopsy; TJ-LB, transjugular liver biopsy.

considered for liver transplant.[6] EUS-LB enables real-time simultaneous endoscopic and ultrasound examination of GI tract and pancreato–biliary system. For example, liver biopsy could also be performed simultaneously for patients undergoing upper endoscopy or EUS for other reasons such as variceal screening and treatment, porto-systemic pressure measurement, or exclusion of biliary obstruction, which can result in increased efficiency while lowering the sedation risk and cost.[7,8] The use of real-time Doppler imaging ensures avoiding blood vessels and large bile ducts during needle puncture, and the use of EUS ensures that the needle remains within the operators' field of view. Generally, EUS-LB is less invasive than the PC-LB and TJ-LB routes, resulting in lower procedural-related adverse events. Compared with the other biopsy methods, EUS-LB offers the advantage of lower postprocedural patient discomfort and faster recovery time (1 hour vs 2–3 hours required after PC-LB).[9,10] Finally, EUS-LB would be the preferred biopsy method in obese patients that may not be appropriate candidates for the PC-LB approach.[11,12] In this review, we provide an update on the emerging evidence, technique, advantages, and complications of EUS-LB for liver disease.

ENDOSCOPIC ULTRASOUND-GUIDED LIVER BIOPSY TECHNIQUE

Several techniques have been proposed to improve the diagnostic yield of EUS-LB (**Fig. 1**). Our preferred technique is the modified one-pass, one-actuation (*EUS-MLB*) wet suction technique with either saline solution or heparin in both right and left liver lobes using the novel 19-gauge (G) core needle. All patients undergo moderate to deep sedation. The left lobe of the liver is accessed with the echo-endoscope in the proximal stomach, distal to the gastroesophageal junction. The right lobe of the liver is accessed with the echo-endoscope positioned in the duodenal bulb and torqued counterclockwise. In patients with altered anatomy such as those with Roux-en-Y gastric bypass, EUS-LB is only preformed through the transgastric approach. The needle is primed with saline solution, and maximal suction is applied via a syringe after 7 cm of the needle had entered the liver under direct US guidance. A rapid-puncture one 7-cm actuation technique is used to sample each lobe for a total of one actuation per lobe. The core needle is then passed approximately 1 cm through the stomach or duodenal wall. The remaining 7 cm of the core needle is passed into the liver parenchyma. Wet suction is used to indicate tissue acquisition into the bore of the needle by displacing the saline solution into the syringe, which then notifies the endoscopist to turn off the suction. Recovery time for the patient postprocedure is minimal, with 1 hour of postprocedure monitoring thought to be sufficient. Once the

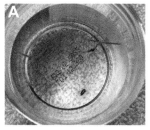 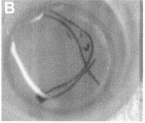 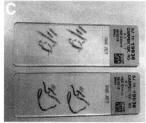

Gross core biopsy specimen   Gross core biopsy specimen   H&E stained core biopsy specimen on pathology slide

Fig. 1. Images of core liver biopsy specimens. (*A,B*) Gross core liver biopsy specimens. (*C*) A Hematoxylin and eosin (H&E) stained gross core liver biopsy specimen.

hepatic tissue is obtained, it is recommended to place the sample directly into formalin from the needle, rather than on a gauze of filter paper (done by some physicians during PC-LB with certain needles).[7] By avoiding placing the sample on gauze or filter paper, there is a decrease in the chances of tissue fragmentation, which can decrease the specimen quality.

COMPARISON OF ENDOSCOPIC ULTRASOUND-GUIDED LIVER BIOPSY METHODS

In attempts to acquire better quantity and quality of specimen, various aspects of EUS-LB technique such as needle type and gauge, needle priming, and the number of passages have been studied. **Table 2** provides a summary of published studies evaluating various methods of EUS-LB.

Needle Selection

Historically, the large 14G or 16G Tru-Cut biopsy (TCB) needles have been used, which were associated with frequent mechanical failure and wide range of diagnostic accuracy (29%–100%).[11,12] More recently, several core needles have become available such as the fork-tipped SharkCore (Medtronic, Minneapolis, Minnesota, USA) and Franseen-tip, three-prong tipped Acquire (Boston Scientific, Marlboro, Mass, USA).

Emerging data suggest that the 19G core needle provides the optimal CPT, TSL, and unfragmented specimen, compared with the other needles. Using this needle for EUS-LB, Shah and colleagues reported a diagnostic yield of 96%, median CPTs of 32.5, and median TSL of 65.6 mm.[13]

When compared with the noncore needle, the 19G core needle has shown to provide a superior histologic specimen.[14] In a prospective randomized trial comparing the 19G FNA needle to the 19G Franseen-tip core needle among 40 patients, the core needle yielded longer biopsy specimens (preprocessing mean 2.0 vs 1.4 cm, postprocessing mean 1.7 vs 1.0 cm, $P<.001$) and more CPTs (42.6 vs 18.1, $P<.001$) compared with the FNA needle.[14] There were no severe adverse events or difference in adverse event rates between the 2 needles. Schulman and colleagues compared 4 EUS needles and 2 percutaneous needles with a variety of suction and fanning techniques and reported that both the 19G and 22G fork-tip SharkCore needles outperformed the FNA needles, and performed at least as well as the 18G percutaneous needles.[15] A recent meta-analysis of 22 EUS-LB studies by Baran and colleagues reported a significantly higher pooled CPT number for the EUS-FNB needle, compared with the FNA needle (18.4 vs 10.9, $P = .003$). There was no difference between the FNA and FNB needles with regards to the TSL (48.9 vs 51.9, $P = .74$).[16]

When comparing the 19G and the 22G core needles, several studies have shown that the 22G needle provides less adequate specimen with higher fragmentation compared with the 19G needle.[17,18] Shah and colleagues performed a prospective case series study of 20 patients who underwent EUS-LB with the one pass, one actuation, wet suction technique using a 19 G needle and reported that the 19 G needle provided a longer core length (2.5 cm vs 1.2 cm, $P<.001$), more CPTs (5.8 vs 1.7, $P<.001$), more total tracts (8.8 vs 3, $P<.0001$), and a longer, intact, fragment length (0.75 cm vs 0.32 cm, $P<.0006$) 18. The only exception to the above results was reported by Hasan and colleagues which showed that the 22G core needle provided adequate unfragmented tissue with a diagnostic yield of 100% for parenchymal liver disease.[19]

Several studies have compared the diagnostic yield of different types of 19G core needles. Schulman and colleagues compared 6 different needles (19G Expect FNA,

Table 2
Outcome studies on EUS-guided liver biopsy

Study, year	Study Method	Patient, n	Approach	Needle Type	Suction Technique	Number of passes, n	Diagnostic Yield, %	Adverse Events, %
Stavropoulos et al,[36] 2012	Prospective case series	22	Left lobe	19G FNA	NR	1–3	91	0
Diehl et al,[35] 2015[a]	Prospective cohort	110	Right, left, or both	19G FNA Expect 19G	Suction (20 mL)	1–2	98	0.9
Pineda et al,[28] 2016[a]	Retrospective cohort	110	Both	19G FNA	Suction	NR	98	0
Sey et al,[37] 2016[b]	Prospective cross-sectional study	45 vs 30	Left lobe	19G Quickcore 19G ProCore	Tru-cut vs Suction	3 vs 2	73 vs 96	4 vs 0
Shah et al,[13] 2017	Retrospective cohort	24	Left lobe	19G SharkCore	Slow-pull	1–3	96	8.3
Mok et al,[24] 2017	Prospective cross-over	20		19G FNB; 22G FNB SharkCore				
Schulman et al,[15] 2017	Ex Vivo Prospective randomized trial	288 samples		19G SharkCore 22G SharkCore 19G ProCore 19G FNA 18G QuickCore 18G Coaxial Temno			85 85 19 46 83 81	NR
Nieto et al,[25] 2018	Retrospective cohort	165	Both lobes	19G SharkCore	Wet	1	100	1.8
Hasan et al,[19] 2019	Prospective cohort	40	Left lobe	22G Acquire	No suction	3	100	15
Bazerbachi et al,[38] 2019	Prospective blinded trial	21	Left lobe	22G SharkCore	Suction (10 mL)	2	100	7
Shuja et al,[29] 2019	Retrospective cohort	69	Both lobes	19G FNA	Wet	3	100	0
Mok et al,[39] 2019	Randomized crossover study	20 patients in each arm	Both lobes	19G FNA vs 22G Sharkcore	Wet	4	88 vs 68	0 vs 2.5

(continued on next page)

Table 2
(continued)

Study, year	Study Method	Patient, n	Approach	Needle Type	Suction Technique	Number of passes, n	Diagnostic Yield, %	Adverse Events, %
Eskandari et al,[20] 2019	Ex Vivo			19G Acquire 22G Acquire SharkCore 19G SharkCore 22G EZ Shot 19G FNA ProCore 20G			superior outcomes i n the 19G and 20Gneedles compared with the smaller-bore 22G	NR
Ching et al,[14] 2019	Prospective randomized trial	20 patients in each arm	Both lobes	19G Acquire vs 19G FNA	Wet	2	Both 100 CPT (2.6 vs 18.1; $P < .001$)	40 vs 35
Ali et al,[31] 2020	Retrospective cohort	30	Left or right lobe	SharkCore 19G or 22G	Wet	2	100	xx
Shah et al,[18] 2020	prospective case series	20	Left lobe	19G and 22G SharkCore	Wet	XX	85 vs 10	0
Patel et al,[17] 2020[b]	Retrospective cohort	135 total	Left or both lobes	Acquire/22G Quickcore/19G Procore/19G Expect/19G	Wet	2	66 46 82 81	NR
Nieto et al,[22] 2020	In Vivo Retrospective	420	Both lobes	19G Franseen vs fork-tip	Wet	one-pass and single-actuation	100	NR
Hashimoto et al,[21] 2020	In Vivo Randomized crossover pilot	44	Left or right lobe	19G Franseen vs fork-tip	Wet	one-pass and single-actuation	100	NR
Aggarwal et al,[23] 2021	In Vivo Prospective Single center cohort	108	Left lobe	19G Franseen vs fork-tip	Wet	one-pass and single-actuation	97 vs 79	NR

Not reported, EUS-TB endoscopic ultrasonography-guided tru-cut biopsy, FNA fine-needle aspiration, FNB fine-needle biopsy, RCT randomized controlled trial, Q-C Quick-Core, 19G FNB needle (SharkCore or Acquire 19G).

[a]Studies by Diehl and Pineda et al. reported the same cohort of 110 patients.

[b]Studies by Sey et al. and Patel et al. are from the same institution and have cohort overlap.

19G SharkCore, 22G SharkCore FNB, 19G Procore, and 2 18G percutaneous needles), and reported that the novel 19G SharkCore needle had significantly higher diagnostic yield than all other needle types in the study.[15] Similar to this study, Eskandari and colleagues compared 6 different needles (size range from 19 to 22G) including the 19G fork-tip and 19G Franseen needles and reported a nonsignificant higher mean number of CPTs for the Franseen needle (11.8 vs 10.4).[20] Hashimoto and colleagues performed a prospective crossover study of 44 patients who underwent one-pass one-actuation method using the 19G Franseen and fork-tip core needles that revealed nonsignificant specimen length differences, but significantly more CPTs for the Franseen needle than the fork-tip (14.4 vs 9.5, $P = .043$), with high histologic adequacy rates for both needles (100% vs 95.5%, $P = .31$).[21] We have compared the performance of the aforementioned core needles between 2 groups of 210 patients and found that the Franseen needle resulted in a significantly higher liver core samples compared with the fork-tip needle (mean core length 3.1 cm, total length 6.5 cm, mean of 24 CPTs, $P<.02$).[22] Recently, Aggarwal and colleagues compared the diagnostic yield of the Franseen and fork-tip needles in 108 patients who underwent EUS-LB. They reported a significantly higher diagnostic yield for the Franseen needle compared with the fork-tip needle (97.2% vs 79.4%, $P<.001$).[23] Franseen needle also demonstrated a higher number of CPTs (9.5 vs 7.0, $P<.001$), longer mean specimen length (15.8 vs 13.8, $P = .004$), and higher percentage of intact cores (75.2% vs 47.6%, $P = .004$).[23] The authors reported that the technical success of the Franseen needle is possibly dependent on the geometry of the end-needle tip and its relationship to tissue acquisition. It is important to note that even the Franseen needle did not achieve the minimum number of 10 to 11 CPTs recommended by the liver societies.

Needle Preparation

Suctioning can be applied in wet and dry fashions. Dry suction is applied using a 10 to 20 cc syringe to maintain suction after passing the needle through the liver whereas the wet suction technique uses the fluid in the needle lumen to lubricate and cause negative pressure to the needle tip before suction is applied either using a syringe or by backward tension on the stylet. A modified one pass wet suction technique for EUS-LB was shown to be superior to dry suction in terms of increasing the tissue yield.[24,25] Mok and colleagues showed that the use of a heparinized needle results in less tissue fragmentation, produced more CPTs, and maintained increased aggregate specimen length and longer lengths of the longest piece than dry methods.[24] We studied the outcomes of EUS-LB in 165 patients who underwent a modified one pass, one actuation wet suction technique (with saline solution) with the 19G SharkCore needle and reported an excellent sample yield with a median maximum intact core tissue length, TSL, CPTs per TSL, and CPTs per sample length of 2.4 cm (interquartile range (IQR): 1.8–3.5), 6 cm (IQR: 4.3–8), 18 (IQR: 13–24), and 7.5 cm, respectively.[25] The rate of adverse events was only 1.8%, which included abdominal pain and one self-limiting hematoma. With regards to actuations, most EUS-LB studies have used from 1 to 10 needle actuations. In the aforementioned study, we also showed that the one pass one actuation technique can provide a sufficient sample adequate to make the diagnosis.[25] Recently, Ching and colleagues performed a prospective randomized study of 1 versus 3 needle actuations for the EUS-LB, using the Acquire 19G core needle biopsy device and reported that the 3 actuations provide longer liver cores with more CPTs than the 1:1 technique with an equivalent safety profile.[26]

EFFICACY AND SAFETY

EUS-LB has shown to produce excellent histologic yield based on multiple liver society guideline requirements. In a systematic review and meta-analysis by Mohan and colleagues including 9 studies and 437 patients, the pooled rate of successful histologic diagnoses and the pooled rate of adverse events were 93.9% (95% confidence interval [CI]: 84.9 to 97.7) and 2.3% (95% CI: 1.1–4.8) with minor bleeding noted as a primary complication in only 1.2% (95% CI: 0.4–3.7) of patients.[27] On the subgroup analysis, the adverse events rate with the 19G FNA needle versus other core needles were 0.9% versus 2.7%, $P = .28$). In our study including 165 patients who underwent EUS-LB with the 19G FNB needle (fork-tip needle), the most common reported adverse event was abdominal pain (N = 36).[25]

ENDOSCOPIC ULTRASOUND-GUIDED LIVER BIOPSY COMPARED WITH OTHER BIOPSY METHODS

Several studies have shown that the diagnostic yield of EUS-LB is equivalent or superior to PC-LB or TJ-LB. Pineda and colleagues compared the diagnostic yield of EUS-LB using the non–Tru-Cut 19G FNA needle with PC-LB and TJ-LB in 110 patients and showed a comparable TSL and CPT count between the 3 methods. In fact, they showed that the TSL and CPT were higher for EUS-LB than either the PC-LB or TJ-LB when bilobar EUS-LB were performed.[28] Shuja and colleagues compared the EUS-LB with PC-LB and TJ-LB approaches in 152 patients and reported that EUS-LB had less complications ($P = .03$) and higher TSL (4.6 vs 3.6 cm, $P<.01$), whereas the CPTs were lower in the EUS-LB group (10.8 vs 13.6, $P<.01$).[29] Mony and colleagues reported that EUS-LB may be more cost-effective than PC-LB particularly when the cost of complications and specimen inadequacy of PC-LB was considered.[30] Finally, Ali and colleagues reported less patient discomfort for the EUS-LB compared with the PC-LB and Hassan and colleagues reported up to 40% fewer postprocedural pain in EUS-LB patient.[19,31] In contrast to above results, a recent study by Bang and colleagues reported superiority of PC-LB compared with EUS-LB. The authors came to that conclusion based on the comparison of the proportion of optimal samples obtained, defined as a sample with a length of ≥25 mm and CPTs of ≥11. Further evaluation of the results in this study shows no significant difference between the 2 methods regarding the number of CPTs, but a significantly higher sample length in the percutaneous group. It is important to note that these results cannot be generalized to clinical practice, as the EUS-LB was performed without fanning or applying the suction, which is known to result in suboptimal specimens, and is not the standard technique used by experts in the field.[32]

SPECIAL PATIENT POPULATIONS

EUS-LB can be successfully performed in patients who have undergone a Roux-en-Y gastric bypass by accessing the left hepatic lobe via the gastric pouch.[33] EUS-LB also can be performed safely and effectively in recipients of liver transplants.[34] A case series published reports of 3 pediatric patients at a single institution who underwent EUS-LB with an FNA needle for elevated liver enzymes, of which all 3 cases yielded adequate CPT and tissue length collection without any technical difficulties or adverse events.[35] Potential advantages to EUS-LB unique to the pediatric population include reducing patient fear and anxiety associated with the TJ-LB and PC-LB as well as eliminating the need for breatholds due to the sedation and analgesia required for the procedure. In general, EUS-LB is contraindicated in patients with platelets less

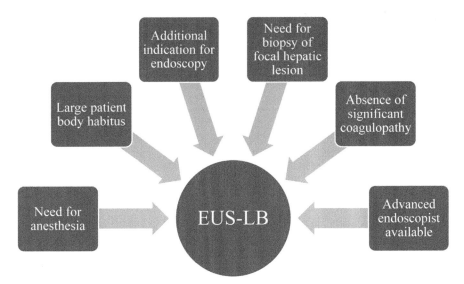

Fig. 2. Factors that warrant consideration of EUS approach to liver biopsy. EUS-LB, endoscopic ultrasound-guided liver biopsy.

than 50,000/μL or an international normalized ratio greater than 1.5 and TJ-LB is favored in these patients.

DISADVANTAGES TO ENDOSCOPIC ULTRASOUND-GUIDED LIVER BIOPSY

One of the main drawbacks to EUS-LB is the relatively complex nature of the procedure and the need for skilled endoscopist.[27] The need for anesthesia and its associated risks should also be considered. Moreover, the EUS-LB procedure is more costly compared with the PC-LB, which can be prohibitive to widespread use. On the other hand, the need for anesthesia might prove to be an advantage in patients who may not be able to consciously tolerate the procedure and in special populations such as pediatrics. If there exists another indication for endoscopy such as variceal screening, then EUS-LB may actually be more cost-effective than undergoing liver biopsy and EGD separately and reduce the risk associated with undergoing 2 different procedures.

SUMMARY

EUS-guided liver biopsy has evolved to become a safe and effective alternative to the traditional liver tissue sampling with several advantages such as the ability to assess both liver lobes, improved the identification of focal hepatic lesions and targeted biopsy, and the ability to combine the procedure with other indications for endoscopy (**Fig. 2**). EUS-LB is associated with less pain and fewer adverse events than the percutaneous approach. This technique is specially favored when patients may require additional endoscopic workup such as upper endoscopy or have an added risk with, or contraindications to, percutaneous biopsy. The additional benefits of EUS-guided portal pressure measurements, assessment of varices, and exclusion of biliary obstruction should move EUS-LB further up the diagnostic approach in patients with unexplained liver function abnormalities. The disadvantages include the need for sedation, associated costs and risks of endoscopy, and training required in EUS. Large randomized controlled trials are needed to directly compare the different needle types and techniques with the aim to achieve optimal technique and procedural standardization. Further research is also needed to further compare the cost-effectiveness of EUS-LB compared with other biopsy techniques.

CLINICS CARE POINTS

- EUS-guided liver biopsy has emerged as an effective alternative to percutaneous and transjugular liver biopsies with comparable diagnostic tissue yield.
- An EUS-guided approach to liver biopsy has several potential advantages over the other minimally invasive methods of liver biopsy, including bilobar access to reduce sampling variability, ability to perform concurrently with other indications for endoscopy and further evaluate surrounding anatomy, shorter post-procedure recovery time, and lower rate of adverse events.
- EUS-guided liver biopsy can provide improved evaluation of focal hepatic lesions.
- The novel 19-guage core needle using a wet-suction technique has been shown to be superior in hepatic tissue acquisition when compared to other needle types.

DISCLOSURE

J.M. Nieto is a consultant for Boston Scientific. I.K. Madhok and N. Parsa have no financial or commercial disclosures.

REFERENCES

1. European Association for Study of Liver. Asociacion Latinoamericana para el Estudio del Higado. EASL-ALEH Clinical Practice Guidelines: non-invasive tests for evaluation of liver disease severity and prognosis. J Hepatol 2015;63(1):237–64.
2. Mathew A. EUS-guided routine liver biopsy in selected patients. Am J Gastroenterol 2007;102(10):2354–5.
3. Rockey DC, Caldwell SH, Goodman ZD, et al. American association for the study of liver diseases. Liver biopsy. Hepatology 2009;49(3):1017–44.
4. Baunsgaard P, Sanchez GC, Lundborg CJ. The variation of pathological changes in the liver evaluated by double biopsies. Acta Pathol Microbiol Scand A 1979;87(1):51–7.
5. Abdi W, Millan JC, Mezey E. Sampling variability on percutaneous liver biopsy. Arch Intern Med 1979;139(6):667–9.
6. Awad SS, Fagan S, Abudayyeh S, et al. Preoperative evaluation of hepatic lesions for the staging of hepatocellular and metastatic liver carcinoma using endoscopic ultrasonography. Am J Surg 2002;184(6):601–4 [discussion 604–5].
7. Diehl DL. Endoscopic ultrasound-guided liver biopsy. Gastrointest Endosc Clin N Am 2019;29(2):173–86.
8. Shah N, Huseini M, Chen ZM, et al. Effective resource utilization with an early discharge protocol for EUS-guided liver biopsy. Am J Gastroenterol 2015;110:S978–80.
9. Takyar V, Etzion O, Heller T, et al. Complications of percutaneous liver biopsy with Klatskin needles: a 36-year single-centre experience. Aliment Pharmacol Ther 2017;45(5):744–53.
10. Sue M, Caldwell SH, Dickson RC, et al. Variation between centers in technique and guidelines for liver biopsy. Liver 1996;16(4):267–70.

11. Dewitt J, McGreevy K, Cummings O, et al. Initial experience with EUS-guided Tru-cut biopsy of benign liver disease. Gastrointest Endosc 2009;69(3 Pt 1):535–42.
12. Gleeson FC, Clayton AC, Zhang L, et al. Adequacy of endoscopic ultrasound core needle biopsy specimen of nonmalignant hepatic parenchymal disease. Clin Gastroenterol Hepatol 2008;6(12):1437–40.
13. Shah ND, Sasatomi E, Baron TH. Endoscopic ultrasound-guided parenchymal liver biopsy: single center experience of a new dedicated core needle. Clin Gastroenterol Hepatol 2017;15(5):784–6.
14. Ching-Companioni RA, Diehl DL, Johal AS, et al. 19 G aspiration needle versus 19 G core biopsy needle for endoscopic ultrasound-guided liver biopsy: a prospective randomized trial. Endoscopy 2019;51(11):1059–65.
15. Schulman AR, Thompson CC, Odze R, et al. Optimizing EUS-guided liver biopsy sampling: comprehensive assessment of needle types and tissue acquisition techniques. Gastrointest Endosc 2017;85(2):419–26.
16. Baran B, Kale S, Patil P, et al. Endoscopic ultrasound-guided parenchymal liver biopsy: a systematic review and meta-analysis. Surg Endosc 2020. https://doi.org/10.1007/s00464-020-08053-x.
17. Patel HK, Saxena R, Rush N, et al. A Comparative study of 22G versus 19G needles for EUS-guided biopsies for parenchymal liver disease: are thinner needles better? Dig Dis Sci 2021;66(1):238–46.
18. Shah RM, Schmidt J, John E, et al. Superior specimen and diagnostic accuracy with endoscopic ultrasound-guided liver biopsies using 19 G versus 22 G core needles. Clin Endosc 2020. https://doi.org/10.5946/ce.2020.212.
19. Hasan MK, Kadkhodayan K, Idrisov E, et al. Endoscopic ultrasound-guided liver biopsy using a 22-G fine needle biopsy needle: a prospective study. Endoscopy 2019;51(9):818–24.
20. Eskandari A, Koo P, Bang H, et al. Comparison of endoscopic ultrasound biopsy needles for endoscopic ultrasound-guided liver biopsy. Clin Endosc 2019;52(4):347–52.
21. Hashimoto R, Lee DP, Samarasena JB, et al. Comparison of two specialized histology needles for endoscopic ultrasound (EUS)-guided liver biopsy: a pilot study. Dig Dis Sci 2021;66(5):1700–6.
22. Nieto J, Dawod E, Deshmukh A, et al. EUS-guided fine-needle core liver biopsy with a modified one-pass, one-actuation wet suction technique comparing two types of EUS core needles. Endosc Int Open 2020;8(7):E938–43.
23. Aggarwal SN, Magdaleno T, Klocksieben F, et al. A prospective, head-to-head comparison of 2 EUS-guided liver biopsy needles in vivo. Gastrointest Endosc 2021;93(5):1133–8.
24. Mok SRS, Diehl DL, Johal AS, et al. A prospective pilot comparison of wet and dry heparinized suction for EUS-guided liver biopsy (with videos). Gastrointest Endosc 2018;88(6):919–25.
25. Nieto J, Khaleel H, Challita Y, et al. EUS-guided fine-needle core liver biopsy sampling using a novel 19-gauge needle with modified 1-pass, 1 actuation wet suction technique. Gastrointest Endosc 2018;87(2):469–75.
26. Ching-Companioni RA, Johal AS, Confer BD, et al. Single-pass 1-needle actuation versus single-pass 3-needle actuation technique for EUS-guided liver biopsy sampling: a randomized prospective trial (with video). Gastrointest Endosc 2021. https://doi.org/10.1016/j.gie.2021.03.023.
27. Mohan BP, Shakhatreh M, Garg R, et al. Efficacy and safety of EUS-guided liver biopsy: a systematic review and meta-analysis. Gastrointest Endosc 2019;89(2):238–46.e3.

28. Pineda JJ, Diehl DL, Miao CL, et al. EUS-guided liver biopsy provides diagnostic samples comparable with those via the percutaneous or transjugular route. Gastrointest Endosc 2016;83(2):360–5.
29. Shuja A, Alkhasawneh A, Fialho A, et al. Comparison of EUS-guided versus percutaneous and transjugular approaches for the performance of liver biopsies. Dig Liver Dis 2019;51(6):826–30.
30. Mony S. EUS Guided Liver Biopsy Is More Cost-Effective Than Percutaneous Liver Biopsy in Patients with Non-Alcoholic Fatty Liver disease (NAFLD). Gastrointestinal endoscopy 2018;87(6):AB326–AB7.
31. Ali AH, Panchal S, Rao DS, et al. The efficacy and safety of endoscopic ultrasound-guided liver biopsy versus percutaneous liver biopsy in patients with chronic liver disease: a retrospective single-center study. J Ultrasound 2020;23(2):157–67. https://doi.org/10.1007/s40477-020-00436-z.
32. Bang JY, Ward TJ, Guirguis S, et al. Radiology-guided percutaneous approach is superior to EUS for performing liver biopsies. Gut 2021. https://doi.org/10.1136/gutjnl-2021-324495.
33. Diehl DL, Johal AS, Khara HS, et al. Endoscopic ultrasound-guided liver biopsy: a multicenter experience. Endosc Int Open 2015;3(3):E210–5.
34. Alsaiari A, Mubarak M, Therapondos G, et al. Endoscopic ultrasound-guided liver biopsy: a tertiary center experience. Gastrointest Endosc Suppl 2018;87:AB339–40.
35. Johal AS, Khara HS, Maksimak MG, et al. Endoscopic ultrasound-guided liver biopsy in pediatric patients. EndoscUltrasound 2014;3:191–4.
36. Stavropoulos SN, Im GY, Jlayer Z, et al. High yield of same-session EUS-guided liver biopsy by 19-gauge FNA needle in patients undergoing EUS to exclude biliary obstruction. Gastrointest Endosc 2012;75(2):310–8.
37. Sey MS, Al-Haddad M, Imperiale TF, et al. EUS-guided liver biopsy for parenchymal disease: a comparison of diagnostic yield between two core biopsy needles. Gastrointest Endosc 2016;83(2):347–52.
38. Bazerbachi F, Vargas EJ, Matar R, et al. EUS-guided core liver biopsy sampling using a 22-gauge fork-tip needle: a prospective blinded trial for histologic and lipidomic evaluation in nonalcoholic fatty liver disease. Gastrointest Endosc 2019;90(6):926–32.
39. Mok SRS, Diehl DL, Johal AS, et al. Endoscopic ultrasound-guided biopsy in chronic liver disease: a randomized comparison of 19-G FNA and 22-G FNB needles. Endosc Int Open 2019;7(1):E62–71.

Endoscopic Bariatric Interventions in Patients with Chronic Liver Disease

Marco A. Bustamante-Bernal, MD*, Luis O. Chavez, MD,
Marc J. Zuckerman, MD

KEYWORDS

- Endoscopic bariatric interventions • Chronic liver disease
- Metabolic associated fatty liver disease • Bariatric endoscopy

KEY POINTS

- Endoscopic bariatric interventions are effective in treating obesity and associated comorbidities, including chronic liver disease secondary to metabolic associated fatty liver disease (MAFLD).
- All endoscopic bariatric interventions should be used concomitantly with moderate- to high-intensity lifestyle modifications in patients in whom conventional weight-loss strategies have failed.
- Gastric endoscopic bariatric interventions, in particular, intragastric balloons, have demonstrated to be effective in improving liver-related outcomes.
- Small bowel endoscopic bariatric interventions have had positive results for the treatment of obesity and associated comorbidities, including MAFLD.
- There is a lack of studies in the setting of cirrhosis and liver transplantation.

INTRODUCTION

The prevalence of obesity in the United States has significantly increased in the past decade. Approximately 30% to 40% of the US population is considered to have class I obesity (body mass index [BMI] >30 kg/m^2), and with obesity on the increase, chronic liver disease secondary to metabolic associated fatty liver disease (MAFLD), previously known as nonalcoholic fatty liver disease (NAFLD), has also increased.[1,2] There is a direct relationship between the pathophysiology of MAFLD and obesity. This pathophysiology involves a state of chronic inflammation and insulin resistance, which leads to an alteration in several metabolic pathways that contribute to adipose tissue deposition in the liver parenchyma. The presence of excess adipose tissue in the

Division of Gastroenterology and Hepatology, Texas Tech University Health Sciences Center, 4800 Alberta Avenue, El Paso, TX 79905, USA
* Corresponding author.
E-mail address: marcobustamantemd4@gmail.com

Clin Liver Dis 26 (2022) 139–148
https://doi.org/10.1016/j.cld.2021.08.005
1089-3261/22/© 2021 Elsevier Inc. All rights reserved.

hepatic parenchyma leads to chronic inflammation known as nonalcoholic steatohepatitis (NASH) and can induce hepatocyte apoptosis and development of fibrosis, ultimately leading to cirrhosis.[3,4] MAFLD has become a leading indication for liver transplantation in the United States.[5] Dietary and lifestyle modifications are the mainstay therapy for MAFLD. A sustained reduction of approximately 10% of body weight is effective in reducing the presence of inflammation in the liver with improvement in both steatosis and fibrosis.[4,5] However, in most patients, achieving this goal is often a challenge, and additional interventions are frequently required. Bariatric surgery has proven to have a crucial role in achieving sustained weight loss and regression of chronic liver disease in obese patients.[6,7]

More recently, endoscopic bariatric interventions (EBI) have appeared as a feasible, effective, and safe treatment for obesity and its comorbidities.[8,9] Several EBI are now approved by the Food and Drug Administration (FDA), and as a general consensus, they achieve greater than 25% of excess weight reduction and greater than 5% of total body weight reduction, and have less than 5% risk of serious adverse events.[10]

Several studies have investigated the effect of EBI on other obesity-associated comorbidities, including chronic liver disease secondary to MAFLD; however, there are limited studies in the setting of cirrhosis and liver transplantation. Therefore, this literature review aims to describe the current EBI and their impact on chronic liver disease secondary to MAFLD.

ENDOSCOPIC BARIATRIC INTERVENTIONS

The current EBI aim to manipulate the gastrointestinal anatomy and alter the physiologic pathways to result in weight loss and achieve all the consequent metabolic benefits. In general, EBI can be divided into gastric and small bowel procedures (**Table 1**). Gastric EBI alter the gastric emptying, alter its accommodation, and improve satiety. Small bowel EBI also improve satiety and interact with bile acid signaling, gut microbiome, mucosal barrier, and neurohormonal signaling. Gastric EBI have been studied more extensively than small bowel EBI; some of them are already FDA approved and have been used for a longer period of time.[11]

Gastric Endoscopic Bariatric Interventions

Gastric EBI include intragastric balloons (IGB), aspiration therapy (AT), and endoscopic suturing devices aimed to reduce gastric volume, delay gastric emptying, and decrease accommodation.[11]

IGB are space-occupying devices that have been FDA approved since 2015. These devices are the most common EBI used worldwide because of their easy placement technique and excellent safety profile. IGB are indicated in patients with a BMI of 30 to 35 kg/m^2 (class I obesity) with at least 1 obesity-related comorbidity and in patients with a BMI of 35 to 39.9 kg/m^2 (class II obesity).[12]

Table 1 Endoscopic bariatric interventions	
Gastric	Intragastric balloons Endoscopic sleeve gastroplasty Primary obesity surgery endoluminal Aspiration therapy
Small bowel	Duodenal-jejunal bypass liner Duodenal mucosal resurfacing Jejuno-ileal incisionless magnetic anastomosis

The American Gastroenterological Association practice guidelines on IGB in the management of obesity recommend that IGB be used concomitantly with moderate-to high-intensity lifestyle modifications in patients in whom conventional weight-loss strategies have failed.[12] The approximate total body weight loss (TBWL) achievable ranges from 5% to 15%. To date, 4 IGB devices are FDA approved: Orbera (Apollo Endosurgery Inc, Austin, TX, USA), ReShape (ReShape Lifesciences Inc, San Clemente, CA, USA), Obalon (Obalon Therapeutics Inc, Carlsbad, CA, USA), and the Transpyloric Shuttle (BAROnova Inc, San Carlos, CA, USA).[11] However, ReShape has been withdrawn from the market (**Table 2**).

The Orbera (Apollo Endosurgery Inc) and ReShape (ReShape Lifesciences Inc) are both silicone balloons that are placed endoscopically and filled with saline (**Fig. 1**). These IGB remain in place for 6 months and are subsequently retrieved endoscopically. A meta-analysis by the American Society for Gastrointestinal Endoscopy Bariatric Endoscopy Task Force reported a TBWL of 13% at 6 months and 11% at 12 months associated with the Orbera device.[10] In 2018, a prospective study demonstrated significant improvement in patients with MAFLD using Orbera. The study followed patients for 6 months and showed a decrease in NAFLD activity score on liver histology and a decrease in liver fibrosis by magnetic resonance elastography.[13]

The Obalon (Obalon Therapeutics Inc) differs from Orbera and ReShape IGB because the device is not placed endoscopically. The Obalon balloon is swallowed as an encapsulated deflated balloon attached to a catheter; once swallowed, the balloon is filled with gas. The balloon is then removed endoscopically after 6 months. Most studies report a TBWL ranging from 5% to 10%.[14,15]

The Transpyloric Shuttle (BAROnova Inc) is the newest FDA-approved IGB device. It is a large balloon connected to a small bulb. The device is unique in its mechanism of action, as it intermittently blocks the pylorus and delays gastric emptying. The large balloon remains in the stomach while the smaller bulb connected by a silicone cord goes through the pylorus into the small intestine. Studies have demonstrated a TBWL of approximately 10% to 12%.[16,17]

Endoscopic sleeve gastroplasty (ESG) is another gastric EBI that has gained recognition for being an effective weight loss procedure with an adequate safety profile. This technique involves an endoscopic suturing system, OverStitch (Apollo Endosurgery Inc), used to reduce the gastric volume (**Fig. 2**). The suturing system uses continuous full-thickness stitches to approach the anterior and posterior gastric wall from incisura to cardia (avoiding the fundus) with the goal of changing the normal gastric configuration to a tubular form, similar to that achieved by laparoscopic sleeve gastrectomy (LSG).[18–20]

Multiple studies have compared ESG with LSG.[21,22] In 1 study, no significant difference was found in the percentage of TBWL between patients (with a BMI <40 kg/m^2) that underwent ESG versus LSG at 12 months follow-up ($P = .21$); however, in general,

| Table 2 | | | |
| Intragastric balloons | | | |
Intragastric Balloon Device	**Characteristics**	**Duration, mo**	**TBWL at 12 mo, %**
Orbera ReShape	Endoscopically placed silicone balloons, fluid filled	6	~10
Obalon	Swallowable deflated balloon, gas filled	6	~5–10
Transpyloric shuttle	Large balloon connected to small bulb	12	~10–12

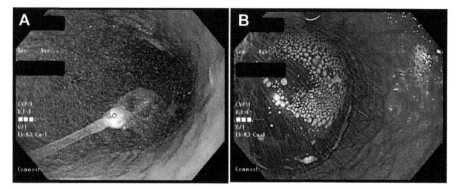

Fig. 1. IGB Orbera placement. (*A*) Unfilled IGB endoscopically placed. (*B*) Filled IGB.

the TBWL in LSG versus ESG was 29.2% versus 17.5%, respectively (*P*<.001).[21] This previous study demonstrated that despite LSG achieving more TBWL in all the cohort, the efficacy of ESG in the subgroup of patients with a BMI of less than 40 kg/m^2 was similar.[21] In addition, ESG has a significantly lower rate of adverse events than LSG. In a 2019 case-match study, the reported adverse rate of ESG versus LSG was of 5.2% versus 16.9%, respectively (*P*<.05).[22] The ESG procedure achieves an approximate TBWL of 15% at 6 months, 18% at 12 months, and up to 20% at 24 months. The most commonly reported adverse events are nausea and vomiting, and only few

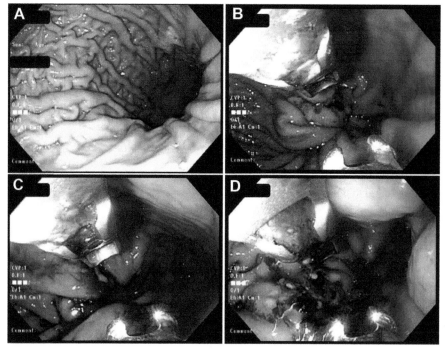

Fig. 2. ESG procedure. (*A*) Gastric body preintervention, (*B*) and (*C*) full-thickness sutures in the gastric body, (*D*) postintervention remodeling of the gastric body and greater curvature.

serious adverse events have been reported (eg, gastrointestinal bleeding, perigastric fluid collections).

Another FDA-approved technique consists of gastric remodeling via a suturing system is the primary obesity surgery endoluminal (POSE).[23] This procedure uses the Incisionless Operating Platform (USGI Medical, San Clemente, CA, USA), a flexible tube, an endoscope, and instruments to place anchors to limit gastric accommodation. This technique continues to evolve (POSE-2), and multiple studies have shown that the procedure is safe and effective as a therapeutic option for obesity.[23,24] No specific analysis has been made in regard to the impact on MAFLD; however, it seems promising because sustained weight loss is achieved in the general population.

The AT device, AspireAssist (Aspire Bariatrics, King of Prussia, PA, USA), is a modified gastrostomy tube that is endoscopically placed. Once in place, the patient is instructed to remove gastric contents approximately 20 minutes after each meal. In order to effectively remove the gastric contents, patients should follow strict dietary recommendations. A randomized controlled trial showed a TBWL of 18.6% ($\pm$2.3%) in the AT group versus 5.9% ($\pm$5%) in the lifestyle therapy group after 1 year of follow-up.[25] In another study, the estimated weight loss reported was 37.2% ($\pm$27.5%) compared with 13% ($\pm$17.6%) in the lifestyle therapy group.[26]

Most common perioperative complications reported were nausea, vomiting, abdominal pain, device site inflammation, and infection. Serious adverse events were peritonitis, prepyloric ulcer formation, severe abdominal pain, and persistent gastrocutaneous fistula once the device was removed.[27]

Small Bowel Endoscopic Bariatric Interventions

Although no small bowel EBI is approved by the FDA, studies have shown that these therapies also achieve significant weight loss, potentially treating all associated comorbidities of obesity, including MAFLD.[28–30]

Small bowel EBI include duodenal-jejunal bypass liner, EndoBarrier (GI Dynamics, Boston, MA, USA), duodenal mucosal resurfacing (DMR), Revita system (Fractyl Laboratories Inc, Lexington, MA, USA), and Jejuno-ileal anastomosis, Incisionless Magnetic Anastomosis System (GI Windows, West Bridgewater, MA, USA).[17]

EndoBarrier (GI Dynamics) is a duodenal-jejunal bypass device that consists of a 60-cm fluoropolymer that is endoscopically anchored in the duodenal bulb. The objective of this device is to imitate the exclusion of the duodenal-jejunal portion in surgical gastric bypass to achieve the same effects on glucose homeostasis and weight loss. The mechanism of action consists of preventing the interaction of chyme to the first portion of the small bowel and upregulating incretin production causing the consequent positive metabolic effects.[28] A 2018 meta-analysis on duodenal-jejunal bypass liner in patients with type 2 diabetes mellitus demonstrated a TBWL of 18.9% with a reduction in hemoglobin A_{1C} of 1.3%.[29] In regard to the impact on patients with MAFLD, a retrospective study showed a significant reduction in liver stiffness after 12 months of EndoBarrier therapy.[30] In this study, liver stiffness was measured by liver elastography on 13 patients with a baseline fibrosis grade of 2 to 4, and a reduction from 10.4 kPa (interquartile range [IQR] 6.0–14.3) to 5.3 kPa (IQR 4.3–7.7), $P<.01$ was achieved.[30]

DMR using the Revita system (Fractyl Laboratories Inc) is a novel treatment in which hydrothermal ablation therapy is applied circumferentially to the superficial duodenal mucosa. The procedure uses a catheter that is advanced over a guidewire endoscopically. Before ablation, the duodenal submucosa is injected with saline to lift and avoid the injury to deeper layers of the bowel wall.[31] Results of this therapy include improvement in insulin sensitivity and better glucose homeostasis by preventing normal contact between the mucosa and chyme. Multiple studies have shown better glycemic control and a decrease in aminotransferase levels.[31,32] A 2019 multicenter study assessing the effects of DMR in glycemic control and hepatic indices showed significant reduction of aminotransferases in patients with MAFLD over 6 months.[32] In the same study, mean fibrosis-4 index decreased from 1.18 to 0.99 (P = .001), providing evidence for DMR as a potential therapy for MAFLD.[32]

Another novel small bowel EBI under investigation is a jejuno-ileal anastomosis performed using an Incisionless Magnetic Anastomosis System (GI Windows).[33,34] This EBI uses magnets to create a shunt between the proximal jejunum and ileum. The magnets are endoscopically placed and self-assembled, creating necrosis in the tissue apposition segments with subsequent remodeling into an anastomosis. Initial studies have shown good results for weight loss; however, as an emerging intervention in the field of bariatric endoscopy, effects on MAFLD have not been reported.[33,34]

IMPACT OF ENDOSCOPIC BARIATRIC INTERVENTIONS IN CHRONIC LIVER DISEASE

The coexistence of obesity, type 2 diabetes mellitus, and chronic liver disease secondary to MAFLD has made EBI an emerging tool for treating these complex conditions. Most studies initially aimed to identify the efficacy of EBI on weight loss; however, more recently, studies have aimed to determine if other obesity-related comorbidities are also impacted after EBI and if they are weight loss dependent or independent.

A 2019 comparative observational study followed 30 patients with MAFLD and obesity who underwent EBI (15 patients IGB/15 patients ESG) specifically measuring the impact in MAFLD using fatty liver index (FLI), hepatic steatosis index, fibrosis score, and liver ultrasound.[35] Both IGB and ESG showed improvement on FLI with no significant difference between them (P = .280). In regard to hepatic steatosis by liver ultrasound, 60% of the patients had a decrease in at least 1 grade of hepatic steatosis.[35]

Another recently published prospective study that included 21 patients evaluated the effects of IGB on NASH.[36] The study used magnetic resonance elastography and endoscopic ultrasound with liver biopsy preintervention and postintervention demonstrating significant histologic improvement. Interestingly, the TBWL did not correlate with the reduction of steatosis or fibrosis.[36]

A noncomparative observational study published in 2021 evaluated the impact of ESG in patients with MAFLD.[37] The study included 180 patients with MAFLD and obesity treated with ESG. Of patients enrolled, 84% completed follow-up at 24 months. Results showed a significant improvement in hepatic steatosis index score. Approximately 20% of the patients showed improvement in their hepatic fibrosis score. Moreover, improvement in hepatic steatosis was sustained until the end of the follow-up period. It was also determined that these patients had an improvement in insulin resistance (measured using the homeostasis model assessment of insulin resistance) after ESG. The metabolic improvements were weight independent.[37]

Two randomized controlled trials comparing the AT device versus lifestyle interventions (diet/exercise) reported improvement in liver enzymes (AST/ALT) at 12 months' follow-up; however, no additional liver-related outcomes were included.[25,26]

A 2021 systematic review and meta-analysis investigated the effects of EBI on MAFLD.[38] This meta-analysis included studies that reported liver-related outcomes after the use of any of the 5 FDA-approved EBI (IGB, ESG, POSE, AT, and transpyloric shuttle). Eighteen studies were selected: 14 studies of IGB, 2 studies of ESG, and 2 studies of AT.[38] The primary outcome of the meta-analysis was change in hepatic fibrosis. Only 4 studies included data on the effect of EBI on fibrosis, all reporting a significant reduction after the assigned intervention.[35–37,39] Secondary outcomes analyzed were changes in liver enzymes, liver steatosis, and liver volume. Liver enzymes were significantly decreased after EBI in 16 studies. Three studies with a total of 147 participants also showed reduction of hepatic steatosis.[38]

Another emerging role of EBI in chronic liver disease is as a therapeutic option for obese patients with cirrhosis undergoing liver transplantation.[40] Studies have reported worse outcomes of obese patients after liver transplantation as compared with non-obese patients, likely related to prolonged hospital stay, longer recovery time, wound complications, and increased cardiovascular events.[41,42] Dietary modifications and bariatric surgery have been studied as therapies for these patients. In general, bariatric surgery carries a high risk of complications in patients with cirrhosis, and treatment should be tailored case by case. EBI are a safer approach; unfortunately, there are very limited data in patients with cirrhosis. A study in 2016 included 8 patients (6 men, 2 women) with cirrhosis that underwent IGB placement for weight loss before undergoing liver transplantation.[43] Seven patients had decompensated cirrhosis, and ultimately, 5 patients underwent successful liver transplantation. The most common adverse events were nausea and vomiting. No serious complications were reported. However, despite the benign results of this study, the safety of this procedure is unknown because of concerns of bleeding in the setting of varices.[43] No clinical trials have addressed the safety of EBI in the setting of cirrhosis.

SUMMARY

EBI are gaining more recognition as feasible therapeutics in treating obesity-associated comorbidities, including chronic liver disease secondary to MAFLD. All of these therapies appear to be safer than traditional weight loss surgery and achieve similar goals. More studies are being developed to examine the effects of EBI on improvement of MAFLD. To date, there are 3 ongoing trials registered in ClinicalTrials.gov investigating the effects of IGB on MAFLD (Clinical Trials Gov Identifiers: NCT04182646, NCT03753438, NCT04230655) and 2 ongoing trials for ESG and MAFLD (Clinical Trials Gov Identifiers: NCT04820036, NCT0406036); all 5 trials are actively recruiting. Because EBI vary on the mechanism of action, not all therapies are expected to have the same effect on MAFLD. However, so far, ESG and IGB have shown good results in both weight loss and improvement of markers of chronic liver disease. Small bowel EBI may have a role in steatosis regression and fibrosis of the liver, because of the tight relationship between insulin resistance and chronic liver disease secondary to MAFLD. Each EBI should be carefully studied with well-designed trials to address the impact on chronic liver disease.

CLINICS CARE POINTS

- Metabolic associated fatty liver disease has become a leading indication for liver transplantation in the United States.

- Endoscopic bariatric interventions that have been approved by the Food and Drug Administration for the treatment of obesity include intragastric balloons, and the aspiration therapy device. Endoscopic sleeve gastroplasty is achieved by using a Food and Drug Administration–approved full-thickness suturing device. All these therapies have shown improvement in liver-related outcomes, including metabolic associated fatty liver disease.

- Endoscopic bariatric interventions should be implemented after traditional weight loss interventions fail and always should be accompanied by lifestyle modifications managed by a multidisciplinary team.
- Endoscopic bariatric interventions have an excellent safety profile in obese patients with metabolic associated fatty liver disease. However, there are no safety data in patients with cirrhosis.

DISCLOSURE

The authors have nothing to disclose.

REFERENCES

1. Hales CM, Carroll MD, Fryar CD, et al. Prevalence of obesity and severe obesity among adults: United States, 2017-2018. NCHS Data Brief 2020;360:1–8.
2. Flegal KM, Carroll MD, Kit BK, et al. Prevalence of obesity and trends in the distribution of body mass index among US adults, 1999-2010. JAMA 2012;307: 491–7.
3. Cusi K. Role of obesity and lipotoxicity in the development of non-alcoholic steatohepatitis: pathophysiology and clinical implications. Gastroenterology 2012; 142:711–25.e6.
4. Friedman SL, Neushcwander-Tetri BA, Rinella M, et al. Mechanisms of NAFLD development and therapeutic strategies. Nat Med 2018;24:908–22.
5. Younossi ZM, Stepanova M, Ong J, et al. Nonalcoholic steatohepatitis is the most rapidly increasing indication for liver transplantation in the United States. Clin Gastroenterol Hepatol 2021;19(3):580–9.e5.
6. Chang SH, Stoll CRT, Song J, et al. The effectiveness and risks of bariatric surgery: an updated systematic review and meta-analysis, 2003-2012. JAMA Surg 2014;149:275–87.
7. Fakhry TK, Mhaskar R, Schwitalla T, et al. Bariatric surgery improves nonalcoholic fatty liver disease: a contemporary systematic review and meta-analysis. Surg Obes Relat Dis 2019;15(3):502–11.
8. Abu Dayyeh BK, Edmundowicz S, Thompson CC. Clinical practice update: expert review on endoscopic bariatric therapies. Gastroenterology 2017;152: 716–29.
9. Jirapinyo P, Thompson CC. Endoscopic bariatric and metabolic therapies: surgical analogues and mechanisms of action. Clin Gastroenterol Hepatol 2017;15: 619–30.
10. ASGE Bariatric Endoscopy Task Force and ASGE Technology Committee, Abu Dayyeh BK, Kumar N, et al. ASGE Bariatric Endoscopy Task Force systematic review and meta-analysis assessing the ASGE PIVI thresholds for adopting endoscopic bariatric therapies. Gastrointest Endosc 2015;82:425–38.e5.
11. Sullivan S, Edmundowicz SA, Thompson CC. Endoscopic bariatric and metabolic therapies: new and emerging technologies. Gastroenterology 2017;152(7): 1791–801.
12. Muniraj T, Day LW, Teigen LM, et al. AGA clinical practice guidelines on intragastric balloons in the management of obesity. Gastroenterology 2021;160(5): 1799–808.
13. Bazerbachi F, Vargas EJ, Mounajjed T, et al. Impact of single fluid-filled intragastric balloon on metabolic parameters and nonalcoholic steatohepatitis. A

prospective paired endoscopic ultrasound guided core liver biopsy at the time of balloon placement and removal. Gastroenterology 2018;154(6, suppl 1):S-1360.

14. Mion F, Ibrahim M, Marjoux S, et al. Swallowable Obalon(R) gastric balloons as an aid for weight loss: a pilot feasibility study. Obes Surg 2013;23:730–3.

15. Sullivan S, Swain J, Woodman G, et al. Randomized sham-controlled trial of the 6-month swallowable gas filled intragastric balloon system for weight loss. Surg Obes Relat Dis 2018;14:1876–89.

16. Marinos G, Eliades C, Raman Muthusamy V, et al. Weight loss and improved quality of life with a nonsurgical endoscopic treatment for obesity: clinical results from a 3- and 6- month study. Surg Obes Relat Dis 2014;10(5):929–34.

17. McCarty TR, Thompson CC. The current state of bariatric endoscopy. Dig Endosc 2021;33(3):321–34.

18. Wang JW, Chen CY. Current status of endoscopic sleeve gastroplasty: an opinion review. World J Gastroenterol 2020;26(11):1107–12.

19. Singh S, Hourneaux de Moura DT, Khan A, et al. Safety and efficacy of endoscopic sleeve gastroplasty worldwide for treatment of obesity: a systematic review and meta-analysis. Surg Obes Relat Dis 2020;16(2):340–51.

20. Sharaiha RZ, Hajifathalian K, Kumar R, et al. Five-year outcomes of endoscopic sleeve gastroplasty for the treatment of obesity. Clin Gastroenterol Hepatol 2021;19(5):1051–7.

21. Novikov AA, Afaneh C, Saumoy M, et al. Endoscopic sleeve gastroplasty, laparoscopic sleeve gastrectomy, and laparoscopic band for weight loss: how do they compare? J Gastrointest Surg 2018;22:267–73.

22. Fayad L, Adam A, Schweitzer M, et al. Endoscopic sleeve gastroplasty versus laparoscopic sleeve gastrectomy: a case-matched study. Gastrointest Endosc 2019;89:782–8.

23. Singh S, Bazarbashi AN, Khan A, et al. Primary obesity surgery endoluminal (POSE) for the treatment of obesity: a systematic review and meta-analysis. Surg Endosc 2021. https://doi.org/10.10007/s00464-020-08267-z. Online ahead of print.

24. Lopez-Nava G, Asokkumar R, Turro Arau R, et al. Modified primary obesity surgery endoluminal (POSE-2) procedure for the treatment of obesity. VideoGIE 2020;5(3):91–3.

25. Sullivan S, Stein R, Jonnalagadda S, et al. Aspiration therapy leads to weight loss in obese subjects: a pilot study. Gastroenterology 2013;145(6):1245–52.

26. Thompson CC, Abu Dayyeh BK, Kushner R, et al. Percutaneous gastrostomy device for the treatment of class II and class III obesity: results of a randomized controlled trial. Am J Gastroenterol 2017;112(3):447–57.

27. Forssell H, Noren E. A novel endoscopic weight loss therapy using gastric aspiration: results after 6 months. Endoscopy 2015;47(1):68–71.

28. Ruban A, Ashrafian H, Teare JP. The EndoBarrier: duodenal-jejunal bypass liner for diabetes and weight loss. Gastroenterol Res Pract 2018;2018:7823182.

29. Jirapinyo P, Haas AV, Thompson CC. Effect of the duodenal-jejunal bypass liner on glycemic control in patients with type 2 diabetes with obesity: a meta-analysis with secondary analysis on weight loss and hormonal changes. Diabetes Care 2018;41:1106–15.

30. Gollisch KS, Lindhorst A, Raddatz D. EndoBarrier gastrointestinal liner in type 2 diabetic patients improves liver fibrosis as assessed by liver elastography. Exp Clin Endocrinol Diabetes 2017;125(2):116–21.

31. Van Baar ACG, Holleman F, Crenier L, et al. Endoscopic duodenal mucosal resurfacing for the treatment of type 2 diabetes mellitus: one year results from the first

international, open-label, prospective, multicentre study. Gut 2020;69(2): 295–303.

32. Van Baar ACG, Beuers U, Wong K, et al. Endoscopic duodenal mucosal resurfacing improves glycaemic and hepatic indices in type 2 diabetes: 6 month multicentre results. JHEP Rep 2019;1(6):429–37.

33. Machytka E, Buzga M, Lautz DB, et al. 103 dual-path enteral bypass procedure created by a novel incisionless anastomosis system (IAS): 6-month clinical results. Gastroenterology 2016;150:S26.

34. Machytka E, Buzga M, Ryou M, et al. 1139 Endoscopic dual-path enteral anastomosis using self-assembling magnets: first-in-human clinical feasibility. Gastroenterology 2016;150:S232.

35. Espinet Coll E, Vila Lolo C, Diaz Galan P, et al. Bariatric and metabolic endoscopy in the handling of fatty liver disease. A new emerging approach? Rev Esp Enferm Dig 2019;111(4):283–93.

36. Bazerbachi F, Vargas EJ, Risk M, et al. Intragastric balloon placement induces significant metabolic and hisotologic improvement in patients with nonalcoholic steatohepatitis. Clin Gastroenterol Hepatol 2021;19(1):146–54.e4.

37. Hajifathalian K, Mehta A, Ang B, et al. Improvement in insulin resistance and estimated hepatic steatosis and fibrosis after endoscopic sleeve gastroplasty. Gastrointest Endosc 2021;93(5):1110–8.

38. Jirapinyo P, McCarty TR, Dolan RD, et al. Effect of endoscopic bariatric and metabolic therapies on nonalcoholic fatty liver disease: a systematic review and meta-analysis. Clin Gastroenterol Hepatol 2021. S1542-S3565(21)00327-X. Online ahead of print.

39. Lee Y-M, Low HC, Lim LG, et al. Intragastric balloon significantly improves nonalcoholic fatty liver disease activity score in obese patients with nonalcoholic steatohepatitis: a pilot study. Gastrointest Endosc 2012;76:756–60.

40. Brandman D. Obesity management of liver transplant waitlist candidates and recipients. Clin Liver Dis 2021;25(1):1–18.

41. Hakeem AR, Cockbain AJ, Raza SS, et al. Increased morbidity in overweight and obese liver transplant recipients: a single-center experience of 1325 patients from the United Kingdom. Liver Transpl 2013;19(5):551–62.

42. Singhal A, Wilson GC, Wima K, et al. Impact of recipient morbid obesity on outcomes after liver transplantation. Transpl Int 2015;28(2):148–55.

43. Choudhary NS, Puri R, Saraf N, et al. Intragastric balloon as a novel modality for weight loss in patients with cirrhosis and morbid obesity awaiting liver transplantation. Indian J Gastroenterol 2016;35(2):113–6.

Moving?

Make sure your subscription moves with you!

To notify us of your new address, find your **Clinics Account Number** (located on your mailing label above your name), and contact customer service at:

Email: journalscustomerservice-usa@elsevier.com

800-654-2452 (subscribers in the U.S. & Canada)
314-447-8871 (subscribers outside of the U.S. & Canada)

Fax number: 314-447-8029

Elsevier Health Sciences Division
Subscription Customer Service
3251 Riverport Lane
Maryland Heights, MO 63043

*To ensure uninterrupted delivery of your subscription, please notify us at least 4 weeks in advance of move.

Printed and bound by CPI Group (UK) Ltd, Croydon, CR0 4YY

03/10/2024

01040483-0016